Dangerous Digestion

CALIFORNIA STUDIES IN FOOD AND CULTURE
Darra Goldstein, Editor

Dangerous Digestion

THE POLITICS OF AMERICAN
DIETARY ADVICE

E. Melanie DuPuis

UNIVERSITY OF CALIFORNIA PRESS

University of California Press, one of the most distinguished university presses in the United States, enriches lives around the world by advancing scholarship in the humanities, social sciences, and natural sciences. Its activities are supported by the UC Press Foundation and by philanthropic contributions from individuals and institutions. For more information, visit www.ucpress.edu.

University of California Press
Oakland, California

Library of Congress Cataloging-in-Publication Data

DuPuis, E. Melanie (Erna Melanie), 1957– author.
    Dangerous digestion : the politics of american dietary advice / E. Melanie DuPuis.
        pages   cm. — (California studies in food and culture ; 58)
    Includes bibliographical references and index.
    ISBN 978-0-520-27547-8 (cloth : alk. paper)
    ISBN 978-0-520-28748-8 (pbk. : alk. paper)
    ISBN 978-0-520-96213-2 (ebook)
    1. Food habits—United States—History.   2. Diet—Political aspects—United States.   3. Diet—Social aspects—United States.
    I. Title.   II. Series: California studies in food and culture ; 58.
    GT2853.U5D86 2015
    394.1′20973—dc23

                                                              2015018713

Manufactured in the United States of America

24   23   22   21   20   19   18   17   16   15
10   9   8   7   6   5   4   3   2   1

In keeping with a commitment to support environmentally responsible and sustainable printing practices, UC Press has printed this book on Natures Natural, a fiber that contains 30% post-consumer waste and meets the minimum requirements of ANSI/NISO z39.48–1992 (R 1997) (*Permanence of Paper*).

For Abbey and Eli

CONTENTS

PREFACE

The burgeoning literature about the history of food advice over the last few decades has led to a greater understanding of American eating. Reading about food has become a kind of obsession for some, and judging from my friends, a caste of college-bred intellectuals, food has taken over a growing percentage of conversations and activities. This obsession about food isn't entirely new. Outside of spiritual subjects, the immigrant grandmother who raised me talked only about her raspberry bushes, her digestive production, and what she paid at the supermarket for things that used to be much cheaper. If we put a listening device on history to see when people talked more or less about food, we could learn a lot about humanity.

This book is a much less ambitious but similar listening device. Part of the listening is to others who have written histories of American food advice. I borrow heavily from these authors. What I have to add is one possible answer to a question that is never quite dealt with in these books: why? Why were the abolitionists vegetarian? Why were the Progressive nutritionists eugenicists? My answer is that it has something to do with the American idea of freedom, an idea that has lit the Modern Age, globally, as both an incredibly successful and a terribly delinquent project. As I note later in the chapters, America is often considered "the original version of modernity." One could substitute "modern" for "American" in much of the book, and I do stray, from the beginning, into that other Child of the Enlightenment, Europe, as both inspiring and inspired by the American idea of freedom.

This book is, therefore, about that group of people who most fervently embraced the Enlightenment idea of freedom: American white middle-

Jean Baudrillard, *America* (New York: Verso, 1988), 76.

ix

class reformers. They are, I hope you will see, a most interesting—and understudied—group of people. Other people do appear, but mainly as targets for white middle-class ideas, particularly the reform project of making everyone "normal" like them.

I was asked the other day if I see my work as "normative" and I answered yes: my norm is not to hold any group's norm as better than others. The history of eating advice, I argue, is a history of people who thought they knew the right way to live and imposed on others their way of life, in order to make them more "free." When presenting the information in these chapters at various times, I've also been asked whether my focus on the white middle class ignores race, class, and gender. In fact, I would argue that this book would not be possible without the work of George Lipsitz, Stuart Hall, Donna Haraway, Patricia Hill Collins, Tomás Almaguer, Nancy Fraser, John Brown-Childs, and others who have given me the ontological tools to look at the white middle class through a feminist and critical race lens. To me, these scholars have not just brought to light hidden stories and silenced voices, they have given the world—all of us—new ways of looking at the world.

ACKNOWLEDGMENTS

This book is the product of three intellectual communities. It began in a conversation with Herman Gray and George Lipsitz, at UC Santa Cruz. I told them I was interested in writing on food from a critical race perspective, looking at purity and whiteness. I had written a book on milk that had basically walked all the way up to the door of that topic, but hadn't opened it. Critical race scholarship is in the air you breathe at UCSC, and I had breathed deeply. But it was Matthew Garcia's book, *A World of Its Own,* and my conversations with him during his visits to UCSC, that made me realize the lack of critical race scholarship on food. Yet, my interest has always been the white middle class, one of the most curious cultures on the planet, and I wanted to look at how American eating had emerged with the growth of the American middle class.

Herman and George encouraged me to apply for a Residential Research Group at the University of California Humanities Research Institute. Groups of scholars live and work together for ten weeks at UC Irvine. David Theo Goldberg, the director of UCHRI, accepted my proposal: "Eating Cultures: Race and Food." This residency gave me the opportunity to focus on a new project away from the cares of everyday life. But more importantly, those ten weeks gave me the opportunity to work with some of the best food scholars in the UC system: Robert Alvarez, Julie Guthman, Kimberly Nettles, Carolyn de la Pena, Michael Owen Jones, Parama Roy, and Sarita Gaytan. We met every week to read and discuss each other's work, and brought in scholars like Matthew Garcia and Aaron Bobrow-Strain, who was then working on his book on white bread. UCHRI likes their scholars to create a product, and ours was the "Food Politics" issue of *Gastronomica,* for which I have to thank Darra Goldstein, who coedited it with great care.

It was a terrific issue, and my own contribution there represents the first glimmerings of this book. Eventually, members of this residency morphed into the UC Multicampus Research Group, "Studies of Food and the Body," which has accomplished so much over the last decade.

My other intellectual community has been, and always will be, the Agrifood Studies Working Group at UCSC. Spearheaded by David Goodman and including Julie Guthman, Patricia Allen, and Margaret Fitzsimmons, the combination of individual talent and the generative process that comes from meeting once a week to share work has produced some of the best work in the field. We produced not only articles and books but also several PhDs who are now major scholars, including Dustin Mulvaney, Mike Goodman, Jill Harrison, and Sean Gillon. One of the case studies here, on the National Organic Standards Board, comes out of my work with Sean. The case study evidence on organic knowledge—the strawberry manual meetings—were made possible when one of the members of Agrifood Studies, Sean Swezey, who was also then the director of UC's Sustainable Agriculture Research and Education Program, invited me to sit in on the strawberry manual meetings. A more detailed analysis of those meetings appears in a book I coauthored with David and Mike Goodman, *Alternative Food Networks*. The organic milk case study also first appeared there.

My third intellectual community was the faculty at the University of California, Washington Center, UCDC, where I found myself, serendipitously, for four years. Faculty from the UC system, as well as local scholars, taught UC students classes during their internships in Congress, agencies, and think-tanks. We also met regularly to share work. It was the most collegial group of people I have had the pleasure to work with, and they had an enormous impact on the chapters as they took shape. In particular, I had the benefit of Amy Bridges's wonderful friendship as well as her expertise in political history. She read and improved the entire manuscript, and we had many lunches where the conversation wandered back and forth from my book to her book on Western state constitutions. Matt Dallek, James Desveaux, Marc Sandalow, and Margaret Howard were constants at our UCDC seminars, and their comments all improved the chapters of this book. I also have to mention Matthew Garcia once again. He was the first person to read through all of the chapters of a very drafty book and help me get from there to here, in part through pointing me to the wonderful developmental editor, Cecilia Cancellaro.

When I arrived in DC, Warren Belasco, Sylvie Durmelat, Psyche Williams-Forson, and others were in the process of putting together a group of food scholars in the area to share work. The Chesapeake-DMV Food Scholars has become a vibrant group, meeting regularly. I was very lucky to share several chapters of the book with this group and to receive not only great input on the chapters but also great companionship from many of its members, especially Warren, Sylvie, and Ivy Ken. I was also able to undertake substantial last-minute changes in one chapter I presented to Karen Leong and the American Studies Department at Arizona State University, where I was visiting along with Don Mitchell. Timothy Lytton's and Keith Schneider's interventions also kept me from making some serious overstatements. You can thank this group, and my newly adopted food scholars group in New York City, Diana Mincyte, Susan Rogers, and Julie Kim, for a much better Chapter 6.

Kate Marshall has been the most patient of editors, as these drafts and versions took shape over the years. Other food scholars in the UCHRI group had finished and published their projects, but I was still struggling to give this book shape. Kate didn't accept anything less than a well-written book, and I went to UC Press because I knew that they would challenge me to do my best work. I look back on my past work as compromises with time, and Kate gave me the time, and the attention over time, that I needed. Production editor Kate Hoffman and freelance copyeditor Paul Tyler added much professional polish to the final manuscript. Finally, my research assistant, Nikita Iyengar, labored diligently over my footnotes. I could not have finished this manuscript without their efforts.

Friends and family also contributed through conversations over dinner or driving (the two places where modern people get to talk). My daughter, Abbey Pechman, realized that the book she was reading for her high school English class, *Their Eyes Were Watching God,* had a lot to do with my analysis of African American food struggles. She went through that entire book and marked food sections for me. I also have to thank the military commissary magazine—the name of which I have now forgotten and which most likely no longer exists—for hiring me to write an article on the Sea Islands abolitionist missionaries for Black History Month, decades ago when I worked as a freelance writer. It opened my eyes to a place and time that has not received enough attention from political ecologists. Finally, two friends of mine, not officially scholars but certainly of scholarly intellect, Patrick Whittle and

Tony Magliero, read through the entire manuscript and made excellent and helpful comments to an author who does not always know how to talk outside her academic circle. They made the manuscript much more accessible to a broader audience. Finally, at the 2014 University of Kentucky Dimensions of Political Ecology Conference, I presented some of the ideas in this book, particularly those on the relationship between citizenship and bodily intactness. Carolyn Finney's critical response prompted me to significantly rethink those ideas which, in fact, better integrated the section of the book on African American struggles over diet, bodily intactness, and American citizenship.

Introduction

AT THE END OF WORLD WAR II, at a small Missouri college, Winston Churchill gave a speech entitled "The Sinews of Peace." Often identified as the event that inaugurated the Cold War era, the speech defined what he asserted to be a new border, one that separated Western freedom from Russian tyranny. Churchill named this border "the Iron Curtain."[1] Yet, his purpose that day was not just to warn about threatening separations but to reinforce protective solidarities: the "special relationship" and "fraternal association" between "kindred Systems of society," especially that between Britain and the United States.[2] The "sinews" were these alliances, particularly through the new global body: the United Nations. In other words, Churchill saw the Free World standing together as a political body, intact and bounded against Soviet tyranny. In fact, in the speech, he talks about the allies as a body, walking together, seeing together. Today the speech is commonly referred to as "the Iron Curtain speech": that is, a declaration of separation. Yet, from Churchill's perspective, the speech clarified the ties that bring a political body together.

Nearly two decades later, John F. Kennedy spoke about an actual physical barrier: the Berlin Wall. Soviets were building this wall between East and West Germany. Like Churchill, he compared the "Free World" of democracy to a captive world behind the Berlin Wall. "Real lasting peace in Europe can never be assured," Kennedy stated, "as long as one German out of four is denied the elementary right of free men, and that is to make a free choice." The boundary not only kept the captured in, it represented a line between freedom and captivity, between force and choice, acting as a bulwark against what Kennedy perceived as the evil system of Soviet Communism, which threatened to deny free choice to the rest of the world.

In the middle of this Cold War Claude Levi-Strauss published a ground-breaking book, *The Raw and the Cooked*, which described all societies, from tribal to modern, through their food choices, using the bounded categories of wild, natural food vs. food that has been prepared—civilized—through human artifice. Soon afterward, in 1966, Mary Douglas published her book *Purity and Danger*, which described how societies defined themselves according to their food choices, choosing the pure and avoiding the dangerous. Both anthropologists used food choice to characterize societies as split between ideas of the social us and the savage other or an untouched wilderness, between purity and pollution, between safety and danger. Both Levi-Strauss and Douglas were hoping to define what was universal and timeless in "primitive" and "modern" societies. But they posed their questions about inside and outside, us and them, during a time when these ideas were very much in the political realm as well. Were these anthropologists discovering the universal social rules, or were they holding up a modern mirror as a way to interpret other cultures?

In other words, the bifurcated view of Western society as a free and intact body that defines "us" against a threatening and dangerous controlled "them" has a history to it. And defining a society by these bifurcations ignores other aspects of that society, the diasporic mixings and confoundings that also explain the Western world.[3] How members of American society set up boundaries of intactness, and then violate that intactness every day, through eating, also has a history, which is the subject of this book.

The idea of Western society as a free body made up of freely choosing bodies began with the rise of the modern democratic state and the Western ideas of democracy and freedom. As this book illustrates, our Western idea of freedom as the purity of free will against a threatening outside continues to dominate our political lives, with serious political consequences, narrating the world as static, unexamined categories. Today, these categories are creating "confoundings": getting in the way of figuring out what we can do about our current, complex global problems—problems that don't fit dualist categories. Yet, as the following chapters will show, the modern Western world has been unable to shake free of these ideas, to create a politics beyond bifurcations.

For both Levi-Strauss and Douglas, the boundary was not an Iron Curtain or a Berlin Wall: it was the mouth. But, like these political boundaries, the story of what people choose to put into their mouths remains, in today's narrative, a story of freedom vs. captivity. Free choice—political or dietary—is based on free will but also on control. Food so easily represents ideas of free will because it is a choice: to put some things in our bodies. But it also entails control: the discipline to keep some things out, to establish boundaries. In this bifurcated world, this choice defines us as "what we eat" and defines the world outside the protective boundary as a dangerous, unruly, disordered "not us," threatening to contaminate the inside, which is pure and free and orderly. So, in a "free world," what Westerners choose to include and what they choose to keep out defines who they are, their identity and social membership. Those who violate this boundary have surrendered their freedom, and therefore their belonging. Members of this society must control the border between inside and outside—keeping the body intact—by choosing not to let dangerous things in.

Therefore the questions "What to eat?" and "How to govern?" have, from the beginning of American democratic society, marched in tandem. Focusing on the American conversation about food, I will draw on American political history, medical history, biographies of nutritionists and gastroenterologists, popular culture and advertising, to show how dichotomous categories and boundary imaginaries have been very powerful—and often effective—ways to organize both physical and political bodies. But these ideas have also locked American society into particular strategies that may not be as effective in the increasingly complex and confounding future.

For Churchill, linking the sinews of Europe and America against the evils of communism guaranteed freedom. Yet, today, in Europe and the rest of the world, American society now often represents the degeneracy of freedom: the spread of American popular culture, the hegemonic global political interventions and wars, the indiscriminate plundering of global resources. Many now see America itself as the "evil system" that has contaminated and captured global political relations. Even those nations not directly affected by direct American interventions still see the vast transformations in their cultures through the spread of American westernization.

The spread of the American diet around the world is an obvious component of this process. When people talk about American food as a problem, they are generally referring to a type of eating nutritionists call the Standard American Diet ("S.A.D."). The center of S.A.D. is meat, made cheap through the industrialization of livestock breeding systems, "CAFOs," often—and convincingly—critiqued as a degenerate and inhumane kind of agriculture. From this point of view, S.A.D. represents freedom, democracy, development, and modernity run amok, creating bad choices that lead to obesity, climate change, animal cruelty, and disease.

It is therefore not surprising that Americans have talked about diet since the founding of the nation. Frederick Kaufman, in his book *A Short History of the American Stomach,* calls Americans "one of the most gut-centric and gut-phobic societies in the history of human civilization."[4] According to Kaufman, our "understanding of virtue and vice, success and failure, has long been expressed in the language of appetite, consumption, and digestion."[5] In other words, the stomach is an important center of American politics, a place to see American "biopolitics"—a "gastropolitics" of "virtue and vice, success and failure."[6] In particular, ideas about diet illuminate the conversation about the moral biopolitics of American reform movements. Beginning with "slave" vs. "free" in the Revolutionary era, moral bifurcations later became the divisions of class and race, clean vs. unclean, Allies vs. Axis, democracy vs. communism, and most recently, security vs. terror.

In November of 1989, the Berlin Wall crumbled, ushering in the eventual end of the Soviet regime. A few years earlier, at Berlin's Brandenburg Gate, US President Ronald Reagan had called upon the Soviets to "Tear down that wall!" He talked about something he had read on the wall: "This wall will fall. Beliefs become reality." Nevertheless, the belief Reagan expressed that day, that "the advance of human liberty can only strengthen the cause of world peace," did not become reality. The Iron Curtain did fall with a remarkable lack of violence, but liberty—that problematic and wonderful idea—did not unfold into the reality Reagan had imagined. Belief, at the time, that the end of the Cold War would create a peaceful and free world was so strong that political leaders started talking about a "Peace Dividend." But this dividend never really came to pass and fully disappeared after September 11, 2001, when the United States increased its military spending in response to an attack within its borders. New threats have led to new bifurcations of the world into those "with us or against us" as George W. Bush put it, with the United States once again dividing the world into the free and the unfree.

Yet, some people began to question this bifurcation, starting with US support of a foreign regime based on questionable ideas of freedom, in particular the Reagan administration's support for "freedom fighters" in the wars in Central America. The idea of freedom became suspect, even as the fall of the Berlin Wall and freedom calls by Vaclav Havel and others reignited a belief that governmental change could bring about a freer world. Instead, new challenges have increased the emphasis on security and exclusion.

In other words, the idea of freedom—and purity—has become only more complex. At the same time, new ideas about the nature of a free society have emerged. This new understanding rejects the idea of bifurcation as the definition of social solidarity and belonging, as well as rejecting the world as composed of pure and dangerous essences—inside and outside—divided by boundaries. From these new social understandings have come new questions about the boundaries previously conceived between nature and culture, civilization and barbarianism, purity and danger, cleanliness and contagion. The last part of the book will turn to looking at the digestive system through these new ideas about nature, in order to better understand the world beyond bifurcations. From this new understanding, it may be possible to imagine new kinds of social reform, to avoid the failures of the past and act in a way that is more effective and, maybe, more free.

This new way of looking at freedom abandons the civic republican notion of citizenship, of the autonomous, intact, virtuous, immune, liberal Enlightenment individual in personal control.[7] Seeing the individual as embedded in "a mangle of resistance and accommodation," in Andrew Pickering's words,[8] describes our current transitions and transformations better than viewing the world as divided into categories of purity and danger and erecting a protective barrier between the two.

Each chapter that follows will illustrate how dietary advice has been intrinsically intertwined with American politics, particularly the politics of reform. Why is dietary advice such a powerful metaphor for political reform in the United States? First, in many cases the connection has been direct: as the following chapters will show, many American political reformers were also dietary reformers, and how they talked about changing diets tells us something about their understandings of freedom and democracy. Dietary advice therefore provides a window through which we can see how reform movements imagined a better, healthier, freer world. Part I of the book will look at four historical eras—the Founding, abolitionism, the Gilded Age, and Progressivism—to show that ideas about good food were imbued with Western ideas of purity, freedom, boundaries, and control. Dietary advice, in determining how Americans should eat, also propounded a particular and fixed vision of how they should live. Ideas about ways of life are attached to particular worldviews, and these worldviews, or ontologies, fix the world into particular categories, or "essences." And such categories then become naturalized: seen as simply what exists, what there is to work with in the world.

Dietary advice is a type of storytelling, and struggles over the definition of a "good diet" are part of the overall political struggle over control of the dominant American social narrative.[9] The word "diet" comes from the Greek *diata,* which meant "regimen" or, more broadly, "way of life." Therefore, subjectivity and ingestivity have been tied together as a solution to the problem of democratic citizenship. Scholars, particularly in the feminist tradition, have noted that politics is embodied and some, particularly Foucault, have shown how ideas about the body changed as ideas about society changed. Examining American political history from this perspective, it is possible to view the history of the good diet and the idea of modern society and the free citizen in parallel.

I term this American gastropolitical worldview "ingestive subjectivity," that is, seeing both the self and society as a controlled and bounded body that makes choices about what to ingest, and in turn these choices create a fixedness, an ontological certainty about what is inside and outside and what to do with it. Americans define themselves, as ingestive subjects, in terms of this control over choice. In a world defined by intact and autonomous individuals, deciding what to put into the intact body implies that Americans are responsible for keeping the danger out, while danger is a threat to that choice, that freedom. As Kyla Wazana Tompkins contends: "Eating threatened the foundational fantasy of a contained autonomous self—the 'free' Liberal self—because, as a function of its basic mechanics, eating transcended the gap between self and other, blurring the line between subject and object."[10] By purifying eating, therefore, one purifies the Self, and fixes the world into two ontological categories: edible and other.

Part I of this book will look specifically at how ingestive subjectivity paralleled different ideas about freedom in four American historical eras. The chapters will show that the metaphor of the body as representative of the nation worked at both a meta- and micro-level, with dietary advice mirroring a larger "orthocratic"—rule by purity—politics. In particular, these historical examples illustrate how American reform movements have practiced an orthocratic politics since the beginning of the nation.

In the first two chapters of Part II, I look at several contemporary food reform issues—food safety, organic food, the Mediterranean Diet—which illustrate the problems of purity politics today and the struggle to create a new kind of politics that is trapped in neither the treadmill of purity nor in the romantic fantasies of a nature outside of ourselves. These case studies show that food reform politics, when trapped in these bifurcations, creates "conundrums": dilemmas that result in an inability to move forward. In fact, in many cases, new policies that attempt to strengthen the barriers between purity and danger only further exacerbate the problems they were meant to resolve, causing unintended consequences that further the food system along the paths that created the problems in the first place. Opening up politics to multiple worldviews through civic processes, while imperfect, impure, and admittedly dangerous, enables better food systems and better worlds.

The focus of the book's last two chapters remains on food, although I turn to the politics of social change in general, and how we can reimagine the world as a better place, without turning to the faulty conceptual tools of purity and romance. In these final chapters, I will describe new ways in which people are talking about the body, as the product of alliances, with nature and with each other. Those alliances, in which we "recognize our bodies as vulnerable to each other," are, says Tompkins, "terrible," but essential.[11]

The problems with the idea of the bounded ingestive body purified by eating the correct food choices might motivate some to wonder: "Maybe we should stop using the body as a political metaphor altogether. Maybe, by abandoning the idea of the body as a political idea, we can get beyond this kind of politics." Part II argues against this response, showing how bodily beingness will always be a part of the country's political imaginary. Also, as a number of psychoanalytic social theorists have argued, how we relate to our bodies will always have something to do with how we narrate the world.[12] But, as Part II will show, the ways in which eating advice fails to nourish indicate something about how our current political solutions fail to make the world a better place. The ideal of a perfect diet—and one perfect ideal of a good society—creates a bifurcated world and fixes this world into two "natural" conditions that cannot be changed, an apolitical world in which, as Susan Buck-Morss puts it, "you fundamentally know the answer to anything, before you even start."[13] If you know the "right" way to live, to act, and to look at the world, those who don't agree with that "right" way are simply left out of the political conversation. And if there is only one way to look at the world, the only way to change the world is through "conversion"—convincing others to believe in the one ideal, by demonstrating to those who don't agree that they are wrong.[14]

Therefore, a bifurcated world that is made up of two categories "known from the start" provides only two political choices: to purify the Inside by removing all that it is not or to reject the Inside as corrupt and romantically embrace the Outside as the Ideal. Romantic reformers have sought to redeem what they saw as a corrupt civilization by turning to an Ideal Outside: nature, authenticity, indigeneity, anarchy, or other forms of alterity. Dietary advice therefore provides a lens through which we can understand the limits of both these choices as a way to deal with our current problems. In other words, a world separated into purity and danger limits social change to either a perfectionist strategy of increasing purification or a romantic rejection of this purity by escape into an uncorrupted, uncivilized, unindustrialized, unprocessed ideal. This kind of bifurcated politics can only follow two fixed paths: excluding some people as unhealthy, disorderly, and undeserving or romanticizing excluded people and their practices as "natural" and "authentic."

Discussing food, therefore, offers an opportunity to engage with the politics of inclusion and exclusion: that is, the ways in which ideas about purity make some people ideal—inside—and others less so. Essentializing the world into the pure and the dangerous tends to justify inequalities as natural, making some people intrinsically less deserving of a good and healthy life because they are deemed "disorderly": less capable of controlling their bodies and boundaries. On the other hand, romanticizing (these same) people who have been historically stigmatized and oppressed is equally essentializing. When Stuart Hall criticizes "the innocent notion of the essential Black subject," he is talking about the romantic embrace of, in this case, a particular racial group for the sake of social reform. Hall argues that when reformers use romantic notions of black subjects, they deny the diversity of the black life experience and instead put a limited idea of that experience to work for the sake of saving the world: "You can no longer conduct black politics through the strategy of a simple set of reversals," he states, "putting in the place of the bad old essential white subject, the new essentially good black subject."[15] In a similar way, romanticizing peasant villagers as timeless representatives of traditional cultures to be saved—and who can save modern society from itself—creates a static idea of who those villagers are.[16] Either path—to stigmatize or to romanticize the socially marginalized—defines both sets of people as static, purified categories. And this political move of romanticizing particular people in their association with particular ideas of nature or history limits the political choices of those romanticized people. In other words, both social reform strategies stultify any real, inclusionary politics of real people in their full experience of the world. Both are politics of stasis, depending on a single vision of one perfect world and change as a purification process toward that unchanging, fixed view of the perfect life.

The final part of the book will examine how we might reimagine bodily relationships to food to create a different kind of politics. By imaging a less purified, bounded, and perfectionist relationship to the world, I open up the body—and eating—to the possibility of relational and discursive knowledge, alliances with people in their messy, complex selves, rather than through either purification or romance. These end chapters can only begin to hint at the potentials for a new politics through this new way of looking at the body and the world, but I hope that this new perspective can point to more productive ways to deal with the complex problems we face today.

THE CHAPTERS

In each era, the metaphor of the body-as-society does a different kind of political work and ingestion creates a different bifurcation between "us" and "other." Chapter 1 will show how freedom became defined, in American political thought, as purity, boundaries, and control. Drawing upon Enlightenment ideas, the American Revolutionary Founders saw themselves as bringing this classical idea back into the material world, as a political practice that broke from aristocratic hierarchies. This has been, ever since, the narrative of American exceptionalism: that we are a country that invented the practice of freedom in the world, and that we have a responsibility to be a model of free citizenship and to spread this model throughout the world. Yet, our ideas about freedom as purity mean that we make the world free through a process of purification toward fixed and ideal notions of freedom.

This first chapter explores the emergence of the autonomous self, capable of free will. The bifurcation of American popular consciousness into a free "us" and a captured "other" started with slavery, and the Founders, many of them slaveholders, defined freedom according to whom they saw as not free, namely their slaves (as well as their own wives, also considered "property" at the time). The Founders divided the world into those who were "dependent" on outside influences—slaves, wives, servants, workers—and those who made choices by exercising their own "free will"—masters, property owners, men. Yet, by that definition, not all men were free: some were under the influence of their own desires, which they were unable to control. The truly "free" were the self-controlled, and food choice became a sign of the virtuous—controlled and orderly—exercise of free will. Chapter 1 therefore follows the development of the modern democratic nation in the Revolutionary period, when the Founders were searching for a way to have a "free" yet orderly society. The idea of a sovereign nation paralleled the idea of the free individual, capable of free will and therefore also in control. Diet, therefore, represents sovereignty through ingestive choice.

Chapter 2 looks at the rise of the middle class and its use of perfectionist ideals to create an idea of moral reform in the early nineteenth century. Middle-class reformers' ideas emphasized highly controlled personal habits and diet as the metaphor for freedom, purity, and control. Against the conservative embrace of purity in terms of tradition and convention—a political move increasingly chosen by the antebellum South as a counter to antislavery pressures—romantic abolitionist reformers embraced the outside, rejecting conventional society as—in Rousseau's terms—"in chains." The abolitionist reformers embraced all they saw as absent from conventional society—nature, vegetables, communal ownership—as a way to solve society's slavery problem. Romantic reformers rejected the inside—the American slave-based society— and idealized everything that it was not, on the path to social and bodily health. Consequentially, free will became self-control against the pleasure of eating rich foods and living luxurious lifestyles. This self-controlled lifestyle defined the middle classes as deserving of a higher moral status.

Chapter 3 shows how the general populace resisted moral reform efforts through the subversive pursuit of pleasure. What early Americans concerned with virtue had disparagingly called "luxury" became a positive symbol of high-status consumption. With the rise of the Industrial Age, Americans struggled over who was to gain the benefits of economic expansion. Yet luxury was only allowable to those who could afford it; those without were expected to remain rational and controlled. The struggle over class control became a racial struggle over the right to a meat-rich diet, as workers worked against the admission of ethnic groups that they perceived as non–meat eaters who would compete against them for a meat-affording wage.

Chapter 4 focuses on the idea of purity as sanitation. The growth of scientific ideas about purity and sanitation gave a new, professional middle class a way to signify their moral status as well as providing them a new place in the industrial economy: as the experts leading society to this purer and cleaner life, and as models of this life, deserving of more. Bruno Latour has suggested that, if germs didn't exist, the turn-of-the-century industrial bourgeoisie would have had to invent them. Germs provided the vocabulary for the creation of exclusionary status.[17] Reformers, for their part, blamed the outside— particularly outside people—for problems that beset American society. Whether they were talking about immigrants in Chapter 3 or germs in Chapter 4, reformers saw the racial outside as contamination and contagion.

The chapters in Part II begin with several "conundrums" of contemporary food politics, to show how the purity and danger dichotomy and the idea of the society as a bounded body harms not just our bodily processes but our political ones as well. The idea of society as a bounded purity paints society as static—inside as orderly and purity as an unchanging ideal—except in terms of becoming more pure. This ideal does change over time as the definitions of purity and danger change, but the idea of the "right" diet remains at the center of social reform. Reform therefore becomes once again an embrace of the fixedness of the center or a romantic escape to what is outside of conventional society. Achieving and maintaining this static society becomes the definition of safety—a safe world is one that is protected from external processes that may contaminate it.

Chapter 5 therefore looks at the current politics of dietary advice, to show that the imaginaries of eating right have led to unresolvable dead ends. Today we see several dialogues around the "What to eat?" question paralleled by questions around how to be "safe" and "healthy" in a technologically, environmentally, and culturally complex social world. In today's dietary reform politics, there is a dominant normative dialogue around nutrition and food safety generally espoused by government actors, often in coherence—but sometimes not—with industrial food actors. There are also dialogues prompted by various social movements, each of which has a different idea about goodness, safety, and social order. Each of these dialogues reflects larger questions about our political choices in terms of how we create our future. They also reflect tensions and conflicts that people have with each other over how they view the world, based on social status, class, race, and region.

In particular, American middle-class reformers continue to embrace self-purification as a way to change the world. Their answer to the question "How do we change the world?" is "We must change ourselves." Like the abolitionists, American reformers are attempting to deal with large, complex global problems through changing personal habits, through an attempt to become pure. When purification does not work, the answer becomes "purify more." This creates what I call a "treadmill of purity" that is, in itself, destructive. Greater eating strictures, purging and cleansing routines, and detoxifications are "orthorexic": an obsession with purifying one's diet, purification run amok. This treadmill of purification by only eating pure food is an attempt to follow an ideal that is impossible to attain. In the same way, reform politics become "orthocratic": an insistence on an unreachable and nonexistent pure ideal.

In Chapter 6 I show how this way of viewing American reform projects as a purification of food and of society—through cleanliness, sanitation, safety, healthiness, naturalness—has stymied the ability of American reformers to deal with contemporary food-safety problems. In the cases of food safety, attempts to build strong boundaries between categories have actually enhanced problems of pollution, environmental degradation, and risk. In the same way, ideas of solving citizenship issues in the United States by building strong borders has only further confounded and complicated the concept of "citizen" in this country. Just as purifying diets have not made Americans more healthy, purification through the strengthening of borders for the sake of security has not made Americans more secure.

In Chapter 7 I begin to describe a way beyond our current conundrum, starting with new ideas about the body. Scientists of the human metabiome have revealed a new conception of how the body relates to, and is part of, the world. The body is not a bounded being but is created by and is embedded in a myriad of other beings. I also explore the new interest in fermentation as a way to reimagine our bodily relationship with the world. Fermentation mixes the world together in controlled but productive ways. It is a dynamic metaphor for a world that can be inclusive yet orderly without being pure. It is also a metaphor for a new politics of practice, of trying different things to see how they come out. It is an imperfect politics because not all ferments yield positive results. In Tompkins's words a real politics of change can be "terrible": frighteningly insecure, beyond our control.[18]

In Chapter 8, I show how these new ideas of the body can help us to see possibilities of social change beyond the system of purity and order. In particular, new, fermentative imaginaries represent a set of alternatives sometimes in resistance to both exalted and degenerated ways of life. We need to move beyond ideas of ingestion and control to more complex and process-based ideas of digestion and ferment. That is, we need to move from being "ingestive subjects"—you are what you eat—to becoming "digestive subjects," immersed in a world of processes that you make and which make you. This kind of politics requires a different relationship to both our bodies and to political society. The idea of the body made up of microbial ferments materializes new ideas about social justice and ways of knowing that see difference as potential, and breaking down borders as the best form of protection. Bringing the marginalized / stigmatized into full recognition therefore becomes the solution to our current problems of sustainability and health and not just a matter of "good intentions" and "the politics of care." Recognition is not a way to prove the worthiness of "good people," to "care" about others, but an essential step on the road to mutual human survival.

Moving our social-change imaginaries away from purification and security may clarify our social concerns and illuminate a set of themes that are intrinsic to a better future. The last chapter will explore this possibility, to lay out ways in which rethinking our food, our diet, and our bodies may help us think through a better politics as well. In this final conversation, "ferment" will represent the imaginary of complex and sometimes controlled but often uncertain transformation. By looking at contemporary fermentive imaginaries, the final chapter will argue that a "politics of ferment" could enable us to see new ways of dealing with the social, environmental, and bodily problems we face today. By changing how we go about knowing ourselves, our bodies, and our social world, we may begin to imagine different futures. We may be able to make things come out all right.

Of course, the body does have boundaries: skin and immunity exist for a reason; it is generally advisable to wash your hands before you eat. Boundedness cannot be abandoned. But, as the case studies will show, the search for freedom as purity is a search for a world that does not exist, because we are not fixed boundaries but embedded in a world of difference that can't help but become a part of us.

Rather than trying to purify food—and the world in which this system exists—we need to muck around in the fermentive imperfection of our lives. People today live in an increasingly complex, entangled, and "wicked problems" world, in which the solution to problems is uncertain, the way forward is unclear, and any decision tends to lead to other problems. In the United States, issues such as *E. coli* O157:H7 threaten, and definitions of "good" and "safe" food only lay bare more complexities about goodness and safety. The uncertainties about purity and safety make where to go from here increasingly inscrutable. In that broader politics, conversations about the creation of a sustainable world are increasingly recognizing that there is no single, perfect answer to creating a better social world for everyone. Science, so often called upon to provide the "optimum solution," is often stymied in terms of which direction to turn. If there are not perfect solutions, either politically or in terms of what to eat, how do we make choices?

Today's world is complex, in ferment, and changing all the time in unpredictable ways. Reformist ideas of purity and control as approaches to "good food" and a "good society" don't work any longer (if they ever did). In fact, as Part I will show, people for the most part did not knuckle under to the visions of reformers and their call for purification and self-control. Business interests, however, benefited from this struggle between reformers and those resistant to the idea of goodness as control, purveying products through which people could get away with their loss of control, such as laxatives and various pills and processed foods for diet fads. These resistant reactions tend to further exacerbate reformers' food moralism. Such purifying projects, however, only exacerbate the problem because they put up more barriers between people with different ideas about both how to eat and how to build a sustainable future.

This book is a call for those of us who have lived according to the orthocratic politics of ingestive subjectivity to abandon this way of looking at the world and of looking at others who do not follow our ideal of a pure way of life. The "we" in this book is therefore the ingestive subject, bound by an orthocratic politics of purity, who thinks that "bringing good food"—and right living—to others will save the world. Instead, sustainable solutions will require abandoning ingestive subjectivity and its orthocratic politics in favor of collaboration with those who have different values, visions, and ideas about the world. Rather than trying to create perfect diets—and perfect ways of life—and then trying to convince others to live according to these dietary and political ideals, we need to pay attention to the social as process, as inclusion, relation, transformation, and connectivity—as "ferment." If purity is a narrative about the safety of who we are and the perils we have avoided, ferment tells us about how we live with the choices we have made, the perils we have chosen, our alliances with those not like us, and the uncertainty of that process. Ferment is the more realist approach to social change. It may involve opening ourselves up rather than protecting ourselves, working with those who see the world differently in ways that will always be risky and for results that are always uncertain. But in the end, we will get to new places that are real, not the pure or romantic world that does not, and cannot, exist.

For those historically excluded from this "we," from belonging in the orthocratic politics of inside, this book recognizes that these boundaries have had violent effects. In particular, the declaration of some as impure and disorderly has failed to recognize, and acknowledge, that other people and their ways of life and eating are deserving of recognition and respect. In other words, purity politics prevents us—all of us, not just the orthocratic us—from moving forward to deal with the problems that face us today.

To do this, we have to rethink our bodies.

PART I

Freedom

Free and Orderly Bodies

PROCLAIM LIBERTY THROUGHOUT ALL THE
LAND UNTO ALL THE INHABITANTS THEREOF
Lev. XXV X.

—INSCRIPTION ON THE LIBERTY BELL

WHAT IS A FREE PERSON? In what way are people "created equal"? And how do a free and equal people create an orderly society? In the American revolutionary era, the Founders repeatedly struggled with these questions. In founding a new and "free" nation of equals, American revolutionaries were surer of what freedom did not mean—the tyranny of monarchy—than how to bring people together in a free society. Once the fight for freedom ended, the struggle turned to defining the outlines of a free and equal but orderly way of life.

"If they were to be a single people with a national character, Americans would have to invent themselves, and in some sense the whole of American history has been the story of that invention," argues historian Gordon Wood.[1] The American idea of freedom and democracy, historian Lynn Hunt contends, required the invention of the American citizen that relied "on an increasing sense of the separation and sacredness of human bodies: your body is yours and my body is mine, and we should respect the boundaries between each other's bodies."[2] Diet, therefore—the choice as to what Americans put in their bodies—has been a mirror of these ideas, reflecting, as John Coveney puts it in *Food, Morals and Meaning,* "concerns about the very moral fabric of our society."[3] This chapter therefore explores the beginnings of American dietary advice as a way to examine embodied ideas about freedom and order in the new American democracy. The Founders struggled with the question of freedom and order, and they did not all answer that question in the same way. As we will see, different ways of thinking about freedom and order also reflect on how Americans have thought about their bodies and their food.

From its beginning, the United States, as a land free from aristocratic author-ity, seemed like "the new Adam of the West, a being unencumbered by the superstitions and fears of a moldering civilization."[4] America was "the world's new hope," leading some to believe that the nation could become perfect, the heaven on earth that would call in the Millennium: Christ's Second Coming.[5] America held a promise of liberty, order, and health, beckoning to the vision of a perfectible life.

American political ideas about freedom and equality developed in parallel with new ideas about the nature of personal life. As people began to practice democratic politics and live this new life of independence, they also began to think differently about their bodies and about the society around them. Human rights in a democracy, therefore, "go along with that bodily separa-tion of a person's selfhood."[6] For the democratic Founders, freedom meant the ability to, in Kant's words, "make use of one's own understanding with-out the guidance of another," that is, to control one's own body without coercion.

This Enlightenment idea of freedom, that each person was an autonomous body, thinking and acting without outside influence, became the foundation of democratic thought and action. The rational citizen was independent, capable of making his own decisions through empirical observation and analysis free from outside influence, whether spiritual, emotional, or eco-nomic. "The ideal of the autonomous individual involved a repudiation of both original sin and subservience to worldly authority, and thus required a reordering of social relations on some moral and voluntaristic basis."[7] The paramount indication that one was "free" was the ability to use one's body as one pleased, controlled by no other person than oneself.

Yet, the dependence on virtue, independence, and character as necessary to a republic of free individuals created a tension between freedom and order. "At the risk of gross oversimplification," David Brion Davis states, "it can be said that the Enlightenment was torn between the idea of the autonomous individual and the ideal of a rational and efficient social order."[8] In particu-lar, the Founders asked: "How do we instill a sense of virtue, or self-control, into free American citizens?" They saw individual self-control, "virtue," as the discipline that would prevent a democracy from turning into a chaotic mob. However, how to instill this virtue into the new American citizenry was unclear.

According to Richard Hofstadter, "The men who drew up the Constitution in Philadelphia during the summer of 1787 had a vivid Calvinistic sense of human evil and damnation and believed with Hobbes that men are selfish and contentious."[9] Yet, their views were not quite as homogenous as Hofstadter states. James Madison and Alexander Hamilton viewed human nature as necessarily self-interested and competitive. "If men were angels, no government would be necessary," wrote Madison.[10] From this point of view, individual freedom became the right to pursue one's own individual interest, and belief in human nature as intrinsically selfish meant that society was built up through the interaction of private interests. In the *Federalist Papers,* Madison and Hamilton therefore advocated for a government of "checks and balances" in which "ambition must be made to check ambition," according a strong role to government structures that would enable people to act on individual self-interest while maintaining social order.[11]

But some Founders, particularly Benjamin Rush, Benjamin Franklin, and John Adams, thought differently: that a democratic society, to be orderly, required the creation of a virtuous citizenry.[12] These Founders held a more Lockean view of human nature, believing that people were born capable of selfishness and self-interest but also of virtue, and that the development of a virtuous character required cultivation and the inculcation of self-discipline. These Founders agreed with Rush that, "Without virtue there can be no liberty." "Liberty can no more exist without virtue and independence than the body can live and move without a soul," Adams stated in 1774. "Only virtuous people are capable of freedom," Franklin concurred.[13]

Thomas Jefferson held a third view: he saw property ownership as the prime motivation for social order, as opposed to the development of a virtuous citizenry or a strong central government. For Jefferson, small property-holding created responsible, orderly citizens. Historian Edmund Morgan's work shows that these ideas were typical of the slaveholding areas of the South, merging the relationship between plantation owners and small landholders into the agrarian yeoman farmer ideology. The South had created order by making it possible for former indentured servants to become yeoman farmers, to create the agrarian society that Jefferson so strongly believed would create social order. According to Morgan, landowners feared the disorder of white, landless people, set free after indenture, competing for land. Moving from indentured servitude to permanent slavery reduced the number of free landless laborers. Less competition for land helped freed servants to become smallholder property owners, "small men" who shared interests with larger landholders even if they themselves owned few or no slaves. Racism developed around this political fix, Morgan argues, by demarcating some people as deserving of freedom and other people as fit only to function as the property of others.[14] By the time of the American Revolution, one-fifth of the nation's human bodies were property.

Northerners like Rush, Adams, and Franklin defined freedom less in terms of property and more in terms of character. An orderly democratic society was built, they believed, on Calvinist ideas of individual self-control, hard work, and restraint—what became known as Yankee virtue. Rather than controlling the bodies of others, Northerners defined freedom as the control of one's own body. Yet, the idea of slavery as control of other bodies meant that the metaphor of autonomy in the North was also defined by slavery: Yankee virtue meant an orderly body, free from enslavement to another but also free from one's own bodily temptations. In the Northern states, these ideas about health as the control over temptation became analogs for a healthy political society as "temperate": moderate in personal practice. A good citizen did not overindulge in pleasure, violence, or luxury, nor was he overly swayed by outside influence. Those who were under that influence— whether at the mercy of their own lack of willpower or confined by their captivity—were not fit to be citizens.

The presence of slavery, in other words, was not yet a contradiction in American society. Slavery helped define the American idea of freedom and citizenship, just as the American idea of freedom as self-control affected the conversation about whether slaves could be citizens if they became "free." Black freedmen became the representative proof of the ability of freed slaves to live in American society, yet the nation did not grant them American citizenship—the right to be considered as able to control their own bodies and therefore full citizens of the American nation—until after the Civil War.[15]

These three ideas of freedom led to very different ideas about how to deal with the nation's problems, in particular, how to make the country both free and orderly. The Jeffersonians advocated for greater access to land and the Hamiltonians trusted in a well-structured government. Civic republicans, however, saw the nation's problems as based in the individual lack of self-control. These differences in perspective led to very different relationships with the popular press of the day and with American print culture in general. While Jefferson and the Hamiltonians certainly represented their views in writing, *Notes on the State of Virginia* and *The Federalist Papers* being two major examples, civic republicans depended on a didactic politics of social change, viewing the fledgling popular press as a platform upon which to exhort the public to practice a more virtuous life. Benjamin Rush's writings represented this kind of didactic politics. His writings on slavery, asylums, medicine, the penal system, and diet represent the beginnings of what would become a constant barrage of exhortations from Yankee moralist reformers on the right way to live.

Rush painted a picture of the virtuous Yankee civic republican that was both physical and political, two goals that he considered intertwined. As a physician, he equated his medical ideas about health as the self-control of individual bodies to Northern ideas about freedom as virtuous self-control. In his essay "An Inquiry into the Cause of Animal Life," he states: "There is an indissoluble union between moral, political and physical happiness."[16] His quest for this tripartite goal led him not only to join in the American Revolution (he was a doctor to the troops) but also, later, to involvement in the birth of many American reform movements. He helped initiate the first American temperance and abolitionist societies in Philadelphia and is pictured on the logo of the American Psychiatric Association because of his work on reforming insane asylums.

Rush derived his ideas about health from his training in Scotland under William Cullen, a physician of the "vitalist" school, who saw the body as discrete and bounded, containing within it two distinct systems: the regulatory system run by the digestive organs and the relational system ruled by the brain. The earlier, Galenic humoralists understood the body as susceptible to outside influences, meaning that "all responses to the environment required a re-adjustment of the humours and of the body's secretions."[17] Instead, in Cullen's view of the body, the brain's role was to make sure that the digestive system did not receive too much stimulation through external inputs such as food or drink. The brain managed the boundary between the body and the world. Overstimulation, in vitalist medical theory, was the cause of much disease, as it led to inflammation of the digestive system. The role of the brain, therefore, was to keep these stimulating inputs under control to avoid overtaxing the digestive system. Health still required balancing, but that balance was a matter of an individual ruled by his own reason to practice "temperance" or "moderation."

Rush extended Cullen's idea of a healthy body to a prescription for a healthy democracy, by linking the rise of a rational citizenship to the idea of the brain controlling the inputs into the body. For Rush, the Constitution— as a product of human rational government—was the perfect mechanism for creating a healthy political body, and the new practices of free citizenship were tied closely both to divinity and to personal bodily health. Celebrating the signing of the Constitution, he described it as "descended from heaven to dwell in our land." This new national document would make "ample restitution" to human nature "for all the injuries she has sustained in the old world from arbitrary government, false religions and unlawful commerce."[18] Instead, "elective and representative governments are most favorable to individual as well as national prosperity," Rush argued, "ordained by God to make men both happy and healthy."[19] Soon after the Constitution was signed, he wrote giddily that this document would bring forth the good American citizen, making it "possible to produce such a change in his moral character, as shall raise him to a resemblance of angels—nay, more, to the likeness of God himself."[20]

Rush argued strongly for republican virtue in his essay "The Influence of Physical Causes on the Moral Faculty." Here he enumerates various threats to the civic virtues of a free life, particularly the overindulgence in pleasure. In particular, he focuses on overeating, which he refers to as "luxury" and to which he ascribes the moral failings of "pride, cruelty and sensuality." Yet, he adds that "the *quality* as well as the quantity of aliment has an influence upon morals; hence we find that the moral diseases that have been mentioned are most frequently the offspring of animal food."[21] Rush was one of the first Americans, but not the last, to consider both liquor and meat as pleasures that enslaved the individual and prevented a life of civic virtue. Because, for Rush, freedom entailed self-control, self-indulgence was a kind of slavery. Order, therefore, came not just from laws, but from inner virtue as well. In accordance with the idea that self-control instilled virtue, Rush was one of the earliest American advocates of the straightjacket, which he saw as a necessary constraint for those controlled by vice and mental disease.[22]

The Northern Founders like Rush saw aristocratic Europe as the antithesis of virtue, degenerate and about to cave in under the weight of vice and "debilitating luxury." "Many concluded that Britain and France and other highly developed nations were steeped in corruption, dependency, luxury and self-indulgence and therefore had to be on the verge of dissolution."[23] When dissolution did occur in France, the Founders shared optimism about the creation of a virtuous citizenry, although the Terror then became an example of what the masses could do if not instilled with virtuous self-control. Rush corresponded regularly with John Adams later in life, and they often communicated their worry about what had become of the nation they had founded. Both saw the country as becoming enslaved to both physical and moral luxury: "not only our streets but our parlors are constantly vocal with the language of a broker's office," complained Rush, "and even at our convivial dinners 'Dollars' are a standing dish upon which all feed with rapacity and gluttony."[24] Gluttony for Rush was the opposite of virtue, both at the table and in the economic world.

Rush formulated the definition of what would become the orthocratic ideal of a pure and orderly society based on personal virtue. He remained throughout his life concerned with how to foster virtuous citizens. Many of his later short popular essays feature particular people who lived long, virtuous, and healthy lives—the subjects of I met a man who lived to. . . stories. The people he praised in these articles were not illustrious, just simple yet virtuous folk who had led long lives free of debased cravings for sensuous pleasures. In particular, he focused on these individuals' health statuses as a sign of their virtue.[25] He also narrated the situations of the less virtuous who, by contrast, led short and sickly lives controlled by pleasure. Letting their vices control their bodies meant that they were not bearing the responsibility of liberty and citizenship.

The virtuous were capable, by healthy habits, of providing their own constraints, particularly in terms of what they did with their bodies. A free populace was therefore one that was temperate—and political rights were to go to those who followed such virtuous lives of moderation. Dietary advice therefore arose with the advent of democratic politics as a way to determine those who were most deserving of rights and privilege, particularly the authority to determine correct ways of living. Like many American dietary advisers after him, Rush saw moderation in food as resistance to gustatory cravings, which he also linked to cravings of masturbation, another bodily activity to which one could become enslaved. Yet, while resisting masturbation generally just meant not doing it, eating as a necessary human activity meant that fostering self-control required categorizing virtuous vs. luxurious foods.

Rush did not advise the total rejection of alcohol, meat, and sweets. However, he did separate out food that promoted independence from food that could enslave. In Rush's most famous public essay, "Enquiry into the Effects of Spirituous Liquors," his ingestive advice involved drink. He listed an ordering of beverages, from good to bad, with water and buttermilk at the top, wine in the middle, and hard liquor at the bottom (fig. 1).[26] However, in his private correspondence, it is clear that "luxurious" ingestion also included

TEMPERANCE.

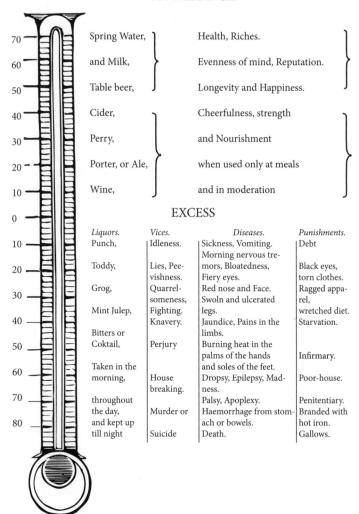

Scale	Liquors	Consequences
70	Spring Water, ⎫	Health, Riches. ⎫
60	and Milk, ⎬	Evenness of mind, Reputation. ⎬
50	Table beer, ⎭	Longevity and Happiness. ⎭
40	Cider, ⎫	Cheerfulness, strength ⎫
30	Perry, ⎪	and Nourishment ⎪
20	Porter, or Ale, ⎬	when used only at meals ⎬
10	Wine, ⎭	and in moderation ⎭
0		

EXCESS

	Liquors.	Vices.	Diseases.	Punishments.
10	Punch,	Idleness.	Sickness, Vomiting. Morning nervous tremors, Bloatedness,	Debt
20	Toddy,	Lies, Peevishness.	Fiery eyes.	Black eyes, torn clothes.
30	Grog,	Quarrelsomeness,	Red nose and Face. Swoln and ulcerated	Ragged apparel,
40	Mint Julep,	Fighting. Knavery.	legs. Jaundice, Pains in the limbs.	wretched diet. Starvation.
50	Bitters or Coktail,	Perjury	Burning heat in the palms of the hands	Infirmary.
60	Taken in the morning,	House breaking.	and soles of the feet. Dropsy, Epilepsy, Madness.	Poor-house.
70	throughout the day,	Murder or	Palsy, Apoplexy. Haemorrhage from stom-	Penitentiary. Branded with
80	and kept up till night	Suicide	ach or bowels. Death.	hot iron. Gallows.

FIGURE 1. A "Temperance Thermometer" originally created by Benjamin Rush in his pamphlet, "An Enquiry into the Effects of Spirituous Liquors on the Human Body," in 1784. This version was published in Thomas O'Flaherty's "A Medical Essay on Drinking" in 1828. The main difference between Rush's and O'Flaherty's versions is that the latter replaces Rush's "Sling" cocktail with "Mint Julep," perhaps a comment on the changing moral status of the South.

too much meat. He included in a long letter of advice to his son, John, who was about to embark on a sea voyage: "Be temperate in eating, more especially of animal food."[27] His own diet emphasized vegetables. One of the founders of Dickinson College, he found it hard to travel to meetings there because there were no meals suitable to his vegetables-and-milk diet in the taverns along the way.[28] Rush represents Yankee democracy's suspicion of pleasure, as well as the consequent motivation to seek and evangelize ways of life built on self-control. Rush saw craving as enslaving, pleasure as suspect, and those who submitted to pleasure as physically and morally unhealthy, yet capable of correction. The virtuous saw it as their duty to instill self-control into those enslaved by pleasure. Often, this craving for pleasure and luxury was associated with ideas of a corrupt aristocracy (fig. 2). Schoolbooks in the Early Republic also tutored children on this notion of freedom as self-control with texts such as: "the sinner has forfeited every privilege of this nature. His passions and habits render him an absolute dependent on the world. . . . This is to be in the strictest sense a slave to the world."[29]

For Southerners, freedom had less to do with virtue and more to do with equality based in land ownership. This agrarian idea of citizenship did not advocate hedonism, but the goal of property-owning was to achieve "comfort." Property ownership would make men orderly in their commitment to their comforts. This ideal of equality among property owners as citizens of equal rank was reflected in Jefferson's discarding of traditional forms of table etiquette in the White House. His institution of "pell-mell" table seating at White House dinners—everyone finding their own seat rather than entering and sitting in the dining room according to aristocratic rank—derived from his belief that democratic manners required all to be treated equally, as citizens of equal rank. Jefferson's conception of an American dinner, which led to the British ambassador refusing to eat at the White House table, was a reflection on his idea of a good American society. Jefferson's White House dinner table was famous for its lavish spread: "Never before had such dinners been given in the President's House," one guest commented.[30] It was pleasure partaken by equals.

As the rest of this book will show, these two answers which the Northern and Southern Founders provided to the question of liberty and order defined the American, and in turn the modern, material body and its relationship to the material world. The Northern orthocratic notion of freedom through control of the bodily boundary separated the world into inner (that which is edible) and outer (that to be excluded). Separating out the world according

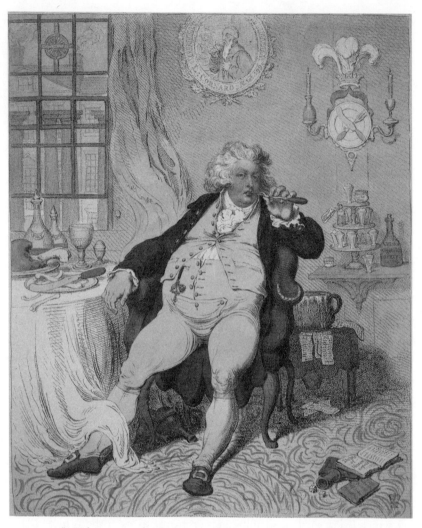

FIGURE 2. "A Voluptuary under the horrors of Digestion," print by James Gillray. The portrait is of the Prince of Wales, later George IV. It is a caricature ridiculing the Prince for his luxurious habits. Courtesy of the British Museum.

to bodily ingestion led in turn to the separation of individual bodies into those capable of controlling ingestion and those deemed incapable. For the Southerner, freedom through property ownership made citizens orderly through equal access to the comforts that property brings. That property included slaves, individuals who provided Southerners with comfort and pleasure.

Both of these politics of freedom justified controlling others, but in different ways. Neither point of view was immediately open to the argument that slaves deserved freedom. Since the opposite of freedom was slavery, a common dichotomy in American revolutionary rhetoric, the fight for freedom from British tyranny meant that Americans "won" their freedom through resistance, a choice of "liberty or death." Because slaves did not—successfully—resist their captivity, historian François Furstenberg argues, they were—like the sinner—seen as not deserving of freedom.[31] For Southerners, slaves as property increasingly became the form of property that brought physical comforts, thereby becoming the source of order and equality for free men.

This tension between self-control and pleasure has, ever since, typified American identity, reflected in both its civic and its dietary conversations. Hamiltonian ideas about getting the rules right and then simply letting citizens make their own choices tends to fall away in these public conversations since, once the rules are in place, there is little to talk about in terms of individuals' private lives. However, the tension between control and pleasure, whether concerning recipes or reform, citizenship or corn syrup, has dominated Americans' conversations about "what to eat" and mirrored the country's conversations about "what to do." The American conversation in the popular mainstream media about eating continues to reflect American tensions about the right way to create and order the nation. In other words, the body has long served as the public imaginary for the understanding of social order in American society, and eating—what Americans choose to put into that orderly body—says a lot about who is in and who is out of that political order.

Rush's political theory of ingestion—that a free populace was one that controlled their ingestion, and that political rights went to those who followed these virtuous styles of life—became the bulwark of subsequent social reform movements, movements increasingly centered in the Yankee North. Creating a virtuous society meant bifurcating the world into free and slave, edible and inedible, sanitary and contagious, purity and danger, us and other, and then getting rid of the bad and keeping it out by purifying society: creating an "inside" and keeping the "outside" at bay.

From the Northern Founders' point of view, those who practiced the self-control necessary to citizenship were free. Those who were legally enslaved were, therefore, enslaved in another way as well, outside the realm of freedom as citizenship. Most early abolitionists were members of "colonization societies" organized to send freed slaves back to Africa. Even those freed slaves who remained in the country were generally not considered citizens, no matter how virtuous their lives. Freedom, therefore, was not just a state of legal being, it was also a test, one that only some could pass.

The following chapters will follow the history of American food advice in order to explore the tensions between freedom and order, pleasure and control, that have defined American ingestive subjectivity. Americans have used food to invent themselves. Eating, therefore, provides a window into that invention.

2

Diet and the Romance of Reform

"WHAT A FERTILITY OF PROJECTS for the salvation of the world!" declared Ralph Waldo Emerson in an 1844 lecture he titled "New England Reformers." Speaking in Boston to William Lloyd Garrison's Anti-Slavery Society, the subject of his talk was, in fact, his audience: New England reformers, whose "great activity of thought and experimenting" had culminated in "temperance and non-resistance societies, in movements of abolitionists and of socialists . . . of ultraists, of seekers, of all the soul of the soldiery of dissent." These "Come-outs," as they called themselves, had rejected the institutions around them, by "a gradual withdrawal of tender consciences." By forming and acting in new associations with new aims, the New England reformers hoped to fulfill American society's potential to become a nation based on virtue. Political descendants of Benjamin Rush and John Adams, these reformers shared a belief that personal virtue—civic republican values—was a necessary part of democratic freedom and order.[1]

But, unlike Rush, who saw American society and its Constitution as creating an environment that encouraged a virtuous citizenry, Emerson's New England "apostles" saw American institutions as decadent and its slavery-abiding Constitution as corrupt. This rejection of mainstream society in favor of an alternative way of life, an alternative that, ironically, fit into an older form of civic republican morality, was part of a larger "Romantic" turn in American arts, spirituality, and culture.[2] Jean-Jacques Rousseau's declaration that civilization kept humans "in chains" inspired the French Revolution and, by the early nineteenth century, was inspiring art that embraced nature and individual "genius" over institutions and authority.[3] American reformers sought virtue in European Romanticism's rejection of its own aristocrats and industrialists and its embrace of high-minded intellectualism and artistic

9

culture. Yet, the American search went further than this, into the realm of spirituality, emotion, and nature. The Hudson River painter Thomas Cole characterized this attitude in his work *The Course of Empire*—a series of tableaux in which a high civilization degenerates, eventually reclaimed by nature.

While American Romantic reformers also held to the view of America as an exception to the problems and issues that challenged European aristocratic culture, they worried about degeneracy in the newer Western settlements and the growing cities: "[i]nfidelity flourished ... and licentiousness bred openly ... intemperance sapped the strength of American workingmen and the saving word was denied their children. Soon atheism would destroy the vital organs of the republic unless drastic moral therapy prevented."[4] For American Romantic Come-outers, working-class decadence—often associated with the rise of the Jacksonian Democratic Party—and national blindness to the injustice of slavery threatened the trajectory of America as a nation built upon shared moral ideals. But in particular they saw degeneracy in the culture of Southern slaveholders.

Southern planters also looked to Europe as the expression of high culture. Yet, rather than the mystics and Romantics, the South embraced European aristocratic ideals of chivalry and honor as celebrated in the novels of Sir Walter Scott. The Jeffersonian notion of property ownership as American freedom became, in the South, a paternalist creed of the plantation owner as lord of the manor, claiming virtues based on honor and chivalry. This point of view did not include self-control among its virtues. In fact, the chivalrous ideas of generosity and hospitality encouraged consumption and admitted pleasure and comfort as worthwhile components of a good life. The struggle over slavery was also, therefore, a struggle over moral culture, between Cavalier and Yankee, and this struggle pervaded American antebellum civic life.

New England reformers who fought slavery, therefore, also sought to form a nation of shared moral ideals. Yet, these ideals were not yet established at the national level. The French aristocrat Alexis de Tocqueville visited America a decade before Emerson's talk. He described the Americans he met during his visit as "possessed by the passion for physical gratification": their lives so centered around the pursuit of "well-being" that they tended to resent the ways in which civic obligations interfered with their private lives.[5] The egalitarian populism of the Democratic Party fit well into the pursuit of a comfortable prosperity and melded agreeably with ideas of Southern aristocratic comfort. Historian David Reynolds, noting the conflict during this era between those striving to perfect society and those seeking to comfortably prosper, characterizes American culture of the time as "an increasingly sharp divide ... one pointing to democratic passions, average Americans, and working-class sympathies, and the other to a more elitist conception of culture, which meant sustaining subtle European techniques while shying away from the vulgar emotionalism and unleashed imaginativeness associated with Jacksonianism."[6] New England reformers, seeking to impose their "respectable" culture on American society, "put a high priority on self-improvement through moral and religious groups—temperance associations, Bible societies, Sunday school unions, and so on."[7]

The ostensible target of Romantic reformers was slavery, but their true target was morals. While most of the American populace in the North saw slavery as a political problem, reformers based their efforts on cognition of slavery "as sin; and to this recognition they bent their efforts." To that effect, Romantic reformers rejected the compromises of politics as morally corrupt. Instead, "[t]heir method was direct and intensely personal. Slave-holding they considered a deliberate flouting of the divine will for which there was no remedy but repentance. Since slavery was sustained by a system of inter-locking personal sins, their task was to teach Americans to stop sinning."[8] Reformers hoped that by "coming out" of established institutions "they would destroy slavery politics."[9] Through their radical rejection of the American mainstream of comfort and seeking prosperity, Yankee reformers sought to create an alternative world in which slavery could not exist. They "sought to purge churches of fellowshipping with slaveholders, and they attempted to persuade all political parties to nominate antislavery candidates."[10] Romantic reform, therefore, became an effort to inculcate a national moral culture, a national definition of a "good" American life.

To do this, the "Come-outers" needed to reject the current degenerate society and its institutions. But, once they "came out," what would they *come to*? What was this other world, this alternative society that would inspire others to follow their lead? And where would this change of heart come from? The answer was a perfectionist ideal, a purification of personal behavior that would lead others to perfection: "The come-outer abolitionists, who eventually took for their motto 'No Union with Slaveholders,' sought an alternative to politics in the command to cast off church and state for a holy fraternity which would convert the nation by the power of example."[11] To formulate this new moral culture, the Romantic reformers turned to the purification of their own personal daily practices, especially their diet.

Through this example, they hoped to create a perfect moral society that, through living example, would end slavery. Yet, exactly what that perfect life consisted of was not clear. As Emerson described it their dietary seekings:

> One apostle thought all men should go to farming; and another, that no man should buy or sell: that the use of money was the cardinal evil; another, that the mischief was in our diet, that we eat and drink damnation. These made unleavened bread, and were foes to the death to fermentation. It was in vain urged by the housewife, that God made yeast, as well as dough, and loves fermentation just as dearly as he loves vegetation; that fermentation develops the saccharine element in the grain, and makes it more palatable and more digestible. No; they wish the pure wheat, and will die but it shall not ferment. Stop, dear nature, these incessant advances of thine; let us scotch these ever-rolling wheels! Others attacked the system of agriculture, the use of animal manures in farming; and the tyranny of man over brute nature; these abuses polluted his food. The ox must be taken from the plough, and the horse from the cart, the hundred acres of the farm must be spaded, and the man must walk wherever boats and locomotives will not carry him.[12]

The link between social reform and personal purity was civic romanticism. Reformers, like the Revolutionary Founders, separated the world into the categories of "pure" and "dangerous." Yet, unlike the civic republicans, who saw virtue in the Constitution, civic romantic reformers rejected the existing social order they saw as corrupt at its core. While following many of Rush's republican precepts about self-control, Yankee civic romantics turned Rush's moral politics on its head. Rush wanted to create a disciplined citizen capable of participation in the main civil society of the Republic. For Rush, the Constitution created a social environment that would enable men to pursue a virtuous life. In contrast, abolitionist Romantics like William Lloyd Garrison rejected the Constitution as the sinful document of a corrupt society because it allowed slavery. By the 1840s, antislavery politicians began to speak about a "higher power" than the Constitution, a major change in attitude from those heady days when the Founders believed that the Constitution itself would create a moral and orderly society. Instead, both political and moral antislavery movements began to see the Constitution as intrinsically enforcing an immoral system.[13]

Despite Emerson's ironic descriptions, these "apostles" were in fact his own when it came to personal transformation in "new modes of living." Reformers were inspired by Emerson's writings, especially on changing the world through what he called "a change of heart." In both "New England

Reformers" and an earlier lecture, "Man the Reformer," Emerson asked his audience "to look to our modes of living" for true change to happen. Combining Emerson with Garrison's radical abolitionist politics, reformers tied personal redemption to social redemption: personal change as a form of moral suasion. While Emerson believed this change of heart came from within, the subjects of his lecture continued to be confident that Rush's didactic politics of public exhortation and moral suasion could influence the hearts of others and thereby create a national moral society.

Yet, New England reformers did not create their new romantic purities out of thin air. New Englanders were Yankees, and much of what they saw as perfect was typical of Yankee intellectual culture that combined the older civic republican virtues with the evangelical spirituality of the Second Great Awakening. Northern, Yankee civic romanticism sought to create an alternative ideal of pure and orderly living, inspired by spiritual awakening, escape to nature, and European Romantic culture. In this process, Romantic reformers, while politically marginal in their own time, created a moral cultural ideal and claimed it as the true American national morality.

Although politically marginal, Romantic reformers spread this ideal through their control of the pen, in that they inhabited that section of the nation that dominated nineteenth-century American print culture. Newspapers from the West and South were "largely sectional in the decade before the Civil War," with only New York and New England "having newspapers that might be called national in appeal."[14] In fact, only the North accepted journalism as a component of civic culture, and the confidence in the role of civic didacticism as a source of political change meant that Yankee civic romantic writing filled the Northern national press despite the fact that it did not represent the mood of the country. In contrast, Southern "[p]olitical influence was not tied closely to reporting" before the Civil War. "Face-to-face politics had always been more important in the South, where lower rates of literacy and lower density of white population discouraged journalists."[15] But reformers, who had a large voice in New York and New England print culture, claimed the voice of a national culture, spreading Yankee notions of moral respectability through these publications.

A large segment of Northern industrialists shared with the Yankee reformers an anxiety about Jacksonian populism and its working-class challenge to the current social order. Both industrialists and reformers shared a patrimonial view of wageworkers, and industrialists approved of the Yankee notions of a moral order necessary for the creation of a new kind of

worker disciplined to the factory schedule.[16] Much of the funding for abolitionist reform groups, including Garrison's paper, came from Northern
industrialists. Therefore, while Reformers and industrialists were at odds
about materialism, Yankee ideology fit well into industrialists' conceptions
of self-control upon which the Northeastern economy could grow. In contrast, the working classes leaned toward the culture of comfort and prosperity and sought it out in the Western frontier. The new urban working classes
in the growing cities resisted the exhortations of their Yankee reforming
neighbors, who made them the local target of moral reform missions.

Yet, one core political belief that Northerners—reformers, workers, and
industrialists—shared was a belief in the sanctity of labor. By the 1830s, the
idea of the independent yeoman citizen that Jefferson had associated with
farm ownership—and which pushed forward the notion of American settlement of the West as Manifest Destiny—evolved into a broader category of
citizenship that still emphasized ownership but had expanded into what Eric
Foner calls "the small producer ideology." This idea of American citizenship
rested on "such tenets as equal citizenship, pride in craft, and the benefits of
economic autonomy."[17] Central to this idea of independent citizenship was
the idea of "free labor" as a "vision of America as a producers republic."[18]
However, as Foner notes, this early nineteenth-century idea of freedom could
not have developed "without a sharpening of the actual dichotomy between
slavery and freedom."[19] Most Americans at this time still fit the definition of
small proprietors, with wage labor generally seen as a stepping-stone, mostly
by younger men "seeking their fortune" through the accumulation of capital
on the way to autonomous self-employment, often on their way West.[20] The
early nineteenth century witnessed the rise of a political party representing
these small proprietors who, eventually, became the political party against
slavery, the newly formed Republican Party that elected Lincoln.

By mid-century, however, with the rise of industrialization, the idea of
a nation composed of small proprietors had begun to fade.[21] The idea of
workers as a class in themselves, rather than a social waystation to proprietorship, began to take shape, and this emerging working class began to gain its
own voice and political place through the penny press and the Democratic
Party, as suffrage broadened to include all white males rather than just
those who owned property. Democratic working-class populists rejected the
abolitionists, the industrialists, and the antislavery parties. Working-class
Democrats had more in common with Southerners and Westerners in their
aspiration to material success and comfort, those characteristics that de

Tocqueville defined as intrinsically American.[22] Yet, the idea of free labor continued to bind Northerners together. Reformers characterized Southern slaveholders as idle, living off the labor of others. For example, abolitionist William Lloyd Garrison derided the South as a place where "no white man will work," because he is too proud to put himself "on a level with the slaves."[23] Work, therefore, to achieve property, rather than property itself, characterized the moral culture of free labor.

Based in this shared belief in free labor as a moral culture, some industrialists joined forces with the moral reformers. Edward Atkinson, an agent and representative of cotton mill interests, who "knew more than anyone else about the financial and manufacturing aspects of the industry," played as much of a role as Garrison or Horace Greeley in antislavery politics, although with much less of a public presence.[24] For example, he helped finance John Brown's Harpers Ferry raid, although he was not named as one of the Secret Six, the group of reformers who were discovered to have financed the raid. As a continuing presence in the economic and reform politics of the United States for the next several decades, Atkinson can be characterized as one of the first to master political influence for the sake of industrial interests. He played a significant role in bridging the economic interests of British and American cotton industrialists and the moral interests of the abolitionists. Nevertheless, "Atkinson's hatred of slavery was animated less by moral certainty or political conviction than by his ardent faith in free trade. In this respect he was at odds with many of his New England colleagues, most of whom believed that cotton profits depended upon slavery. Atkinson believed that cotton could be cultivated by white and free blacks 'with perfect ease and safety.'"[25] Atkinson published an article that analyzed the U.S. census to show that cotton was vastly underproduced in the slave states and that more and more cotton was being grown by free landholders in Tennessee and Texas. He cited these facts as proof that cotton could be grown more efficiently under a free labor regime. Atkinson's arguments were widely publicized and Greeley, publisher of the antislavery *New York Tribune*, quoted freely from Atkinson's economic arguments against slavery.

The abolitionists, however, rejected antislavery political parties in the same way they rejected conventional religious institutions—none were pure enough. They also rejected the more common view of slavery as a political and economic problem. To abolitionists, framing the antislavery narrative in terms of politics and economics was sinful in itself; slavery was sin and the only solution was a moral crusade. For the abolitionists, the answer was through a didactic politics that would purify the American populace into an Emersonian "change of heart," bringing citizens to the idea that slavery should be immediately abolished.

As Emerson described in his lecture, abolitionist reformers provided themselves as examples in the practice of purified lifestyles. They tended to reject both meat and alcohol in an era when Americans consumed both heavily. Many were followers of vegetarian advocate Sylvester Graham— "Grahamites"—who pledged to eat no meat and only ate bread made with whole-wheat "graham" flour. In the 1830s, Graham—who began as a temperance lecturer—toured the North, propounding publicly the benefits of a diet of vegetables and unyeasted bread of unbolted or "graham" flour. Many abolitionists adhered to Graham's precepts, including Thoreau, who at Walden described making bread without yeast. Temperance, abolitionism, and Grahamite vegetarianism went hand in hand.

Graham was therefore emblematic of the era's reformers: an apostle evangelizing a vision of how purification of self could purify society and thereby save it.[26] Graham believed that self-purification was the solution to problems such as the spate of cholera epidemics, which he blamed on luxurious living: "only by such severe and awful retributions from the violated laws of nature, have mankind been induced to pause from their sensual excesses, and investigate even the most obvious relations between their habits and their sufferings."[27] Yankee morality combined Graham's ideas about physical health as self-purification and Northern moral precepts of self-control.

While not strictly or always vegetarians, Emerson and other transcendentalists shared with the New England reformers a rejection of materialism, which included strictures against consuming luxurious food: "It is for cake that we run in debt," wrote Emerson. "We dare not trust our wit in making our house pleasant to our friend, and so we buy ice-creams."[28] Luxurious food, for Emerson, was a sign of conformity and, like Rush, he saw it as an enslavement to material pleasures. Yet, unlike Rush, who envisioned a temperate life as creating a good society, Emerson saw the rejection of luxurious foods as a way to escape the bonds of social expectations. Reformers saw it as both, equating a romantic rejection of corrupt society with an embrace of self-control.

Jacksonian popular newspapers resisted the exhortations of didactic politics. The slavery-tolerant *New York Herald* parodied abolitionists for their vegetarian leanings. In particular, the *Herald* targeted Greeley, the editor of its competitor, the *New York Tribune,* as "the king of the vegetarians." Horace

Greeley was never much of a vegetarian. "The nation's most loved, hated and widely read newspaper editor" frequented Delmonico's restaurant and in his autobiography he talks about his love of a good steak.[29] However, the *Tribune* was respectful of civic romantic reformers and accepted its antislavery stance. In addition, Greeley wrote positively about vegetarianism. Tellingly, the *Herald* often attacked Greeley's strong support of the Civil War by attacking his ostensible vegetarian diet. Describing Greeley as a "teetotaler and a vegetarian," the paper vilified Greeley as a warmonger, and furthermore as a hypocrite for not fighting himself, while pushing others into battle, turning him "from a vegetarian . . . into an ogre, eating human flesh."[30] The *Herald's* constant linkage between support for the war and against slavery with vegetarianism "thus framed abolitionists and vegetarians as elitists, philosophers out of touch with both the general public and Union fighting forces."[31]

Yet, Greeley's paper, nicknamed "the Great Moral Organ," had the country's largest national subscription and was the first of the penny press to reject populist sensationalism in favor of a moral mouthpiece, espousing various Whig reforms such as vegetarianism, temperance, and especially abolition. Greeley's popularity was based not simply on his moral stances but also on his representation as a "self-made man" and, as such, a follower of the free labor creed that condemned Southern slavery. Yet, wageworkers were largely readers of the more populist and sensationalist *Herald* that attacked Greeley as weakened by his supposed vegetarian diet and living on the blood of dead working-class soldiers. The *Herald,* representing popular sentiment against the war among the city's working class, taunted Greeley about his eating habits and his views: while "the smell of roast meat or the sight of gravy made him sick at his stomach," the *Herald* claimed, this "monster, ogre, ghoul, will soon feast his last upon Union blood and national spoils."[32]

The *Herald* represented the average American citizen, generally urban and working class, who rejected the civic didactic exhortations of the Yankee reformers. In fact, many of the main voices of Northern print culture accepted slavery as necessary for maintaining the Union. The most influential voices of the period—such as Sarah Josepha Hale, editor of *Godey's Lady's Book,* and Daniel Webster—either avoided the slavery issue or emphasized the Union over abolition. Not only were abolitionists marginalized by majority pro-Union sentiments; they were also divided from the antislavery press that supported political parties—rather than moral conversion—as a way toward Emancipation. Many abolitionists therefore abjured both meat-eating and political institutions as corrupt practices.

In their rejection of political institutions, moral reformers romantically embraced everything the rapidly industrializing society was not: spiritual revelation, nature, European intellectual culture, and the old civic republican ideas of virtue abandoned by the Jacksonians. Reformers envisioned creating a new and pure way of life and then going out to evangelize, to spread the model of this good life through books, articles, and lectures. The focus was on changing the greater public consciousness—the change of heart necessary for the creation of a new world. They sought to bring others from artificiality to authenticity, from the degraded city to the purity of nature, and away from the materialism of the emerging industrial society. In their search for new ways of life, Yankee reformers found particular inspiration for their visions of a good society in three Romantic sources: revelation, nature, and Europe.

Revelation

While it was Garrison who ignited the moral crusade against slavery, it was Charles Grandison Finney who inspired Yankee faith in the creation of a perfect society. For the up-and-coming middle class who wanted to separate themselves from the masses and join the ranks of the virtuous, Finney and Graham's moral stands created a powerful semiotics of social deservedness through displays of self-discipline.[33] Finney was the Second Great Awakening's chief evangelist, traveling to the same towns as Emerson, Garrison, and other reformers, but often forced to preach in tent revivals outside of those towns in order to handle the crowds that flocked to him. Finney espoused a form of redemption that challenged the old Calvinist patriarchal notions of predestination and fate, instead arguing for a new faith in the ability of the individual to save him- or herself through confession and conversion—a more religious version of Emerson's "change of heart." The converted not only could perfect themselves, they could also create a new and perfect world in which "[s]alvation, however variously defined, lay open to everyone. Sin was voluntary: men were not helpless and depraved by nature but free agents and potential powers for good. Sin could be reduced to the selfish preferences of individuals, and social evils, in turn, to collective sins which, once acknowledged, could be rooted out."[34]

Many abolitionists were inspired as much by Finney's Perfectionism as by Emerson's Transcendentalism or Graham's vegetarianism. This "romantic faith in perfectibility, originally confined by religious institutions, overflow[ed] these barriers and spread across the surface of society, seeping into politics and culture."[35] The Erie Canal was a 300-mile monument to this new human faith in improvement, allowing goods to be carried from New York City to Buffalo and beyond. It changed the landscape of upstate New York, and those who lived there were inspired by this human ability to change the world. Finney termed the canal region "the Burned-Over District" due to the fires of redemption burning brightly throughout this area.

The rejection of established religious institutions and embrace of evangelism meant that Romantic reformers relied on a "visionary culture," one in which individual divine revelation held as much authority as any institutional religious authority.[36] Reform associations—for temperance, against slavery, and advocating various changes in modes of life, including vegetarianism—often followed the style of the evangelical meeting, including individual public confession and a membership pledge. Much like the confession and pledge practices that evangelical preacher Charles Grandison Finney brought to the lecture circuit, the individual confession and pledge merged self-reform and spiritual salvation, often leaving them susceptible to what contemporaries called "enthusiasms." One historian called this era "the Stammering Century," where, at revival meetings, participants "shrieked and groaned and fallen into epilepsy before the revivalist ... rose and announced that God had spoken to them, predicted the death of individuals, the destruction of cities, and the damnation of all who did not repent and accept Christ."[37] Some heard voices; others were visited by angels. Finney himself never claimed to have seen an angel, but he did describe seeing a "bright light" in 1829, which prompted him to leave lawyering and take up the life of a preacher.[38]

It is not surprising, then, that some dietary reformers in this period, like the preachers of the day, narrated their personal transformation as a direct experience with the divine. Many stories of dietary reform begin with visionary narratives. Joseph Smith, for example, received dietary advice from the Angel Moroni, who handed Smith not just the Golden Tablets but a set of instructions on good living called the Word of Wisdom. The advice was much like the dietary advice of the day, advising moderation, especially in consuming meat. Ellen G. White combined Grahamite food prohibition with angelic visions to provide the spiritual and ingestive foundations of the Seventh-day Adventists: the avoidance of meat, alcohol, caffeine, tobacco, salt, stuffy rooms, and doctors.[39] Originally a follower of millenarian William Miller, who predicted the end of the world on various days in 1844, she turned

Millerite followers away from preparing for the apocalypse and toward temperate living and sabbatarianism after "the Great Disappointment": the failure of the world to end as predicted by Miller. Even while attention to daily health habits and dietary reform abated amid the more important health issues of Civil War slaughter and disease, White continued to preach a dietary gospel. Her first vegetarian visions arrived during the Battle of Vicksburg, and an edition of her collection of visions, *Spiritual Gifts,* was published during Sherman's march to Atlanta. To White, intemperance, not war, was the greatest human downfall, and God's will was not victory over the South but victory over one's bodily habits.[40]

Although he relied more on scientific authority than the Bible, Graham began his career as an ordained minister in the Presbyterian Church. Reformers took his word as received dietary prophecy and spread this divine dietary vision among those suffering from the sins of digestive moral degeneracy. Oneida, like many utopian spiritual communities, also followed vegetarian principles based largely on Graham. By the 1840s, even the Shaker communities—which had been founded decades earlier on Ann Lee's visions of discipline through celibacy, not diet—became increasingly vegetarian through the influence of Graham. His forceful arguments that spicy foods encouraged lust were enough for the celibate Shakers to sign on to his diet. In addition, certain members reported receiving visions of "Mother Ann" returning in spirit to espouse various dietary restrictions.[41]

When direct divine advice was missing, food reformers like Graham used a peculiar semi-scientific deism as their method, counting on the Bible to provide them with scientific data about a better future. Food reformer Robert Hartley interpreted God's preference of Abel over Cain as indicating that humans should drink milk. Hartley combined this biblical interpretation with new European science about the nature of digestion in his fight against city "swill milk" dairies, where cows ate brewery waste and lived in horribly unsanitary conditions.[42] But Hartley's inspiration went beyond biblical interpretation. The opening scene in his biography—written by his son—includes a vision narrative: the apparition of an angel who told him to quit his job as a factory manager and pursue a soul-saving life in New York City.[43]

Evangelicals therefore proposed spiritual and physical salvation through dietary reform. Finney attempted to feed Oberlin College students a Grahamite diet, only to prompt an early example of that now-venerable institution: the college protest. Whether spiritual or dietary, a didactic politics of conversion became the major reform strategy, a strategy dependent on bifurcating the world and then convincing the "bad" side to be "good."

While their numbers were small, the Grahamites were closely knit and dedicated to a range of reforms. One resident described a New York Grahamite boardinghouse as "not only Grahamites but Garrisonites—not only reformers in diet, but radicalists in Politics. Such a knot of Abolitionists I never before fell in with."[44] All through the Northern states, abolitionists met in these vegetarian boardinghouses, eating their meatless dinners while speaking of the evils of slavery. Horace Greeley and William Lloyd Garrison dined together at a New York Grahamite house. The major abolitionists who were also Grahamites (some of them, like Greeley and Garrison, more allies than practitioners) included Theodore Weld and the Grimke sisters, William and his brother Bronson Alcott, the Tappan Brothers, and Gerrit Smith, one of the "Secret Six" who financed John Brown's raid at Harpers Ferry. The dinner table at Grahamite boardinghouses became a favorite meeting place for all the active reform movements. Those who supported abolition and temperance, and who opposed tobacco and masturbation, constantly swapped ideas at Grahamite tables.

While Garrison was not committed to vegetarianism, his famous essay, "The War—Its Cause and Cure," published in his abolitionist newspaper *The Liberator* at the beginning of the Civil War, argues that the war must end with Emancipation and uses diet as a metaphor to make his point. Using a food metaphor, he argues that the Constitution provided food for slavery: "nourishment, defense and security from the whole body politic." Garrison warns that this Constitutional nourishment must be removed from the American diet. At the end of the essay, he quotes a passage from the Bible rich in food metaphors. Until slaves were delivered "out of the hands of the oppressor": "the sword of the Lord shall devour from the one end of the land to the other: no flesh shall have peace."[45] The Constitution fed slavery, while devouring the body of the country as a whole. Only by removing slavery from the American diet would the political body have peace. These biblical quotes echoed the vegetarian testimonials of the day, in which people spoke of physical distress until they removed meat from the diet, often described as both a physical and spiritual awakening.

Rochester, New York, which was transformed into a boomtown by the opening of the Erie Canal in 1823, illustrates the combined influences of visionary, romantic, and vegetarian reform movements. With Rochester located squarely in the center of the Burned-Over District, Finney preached there often, as did Graham, Emerson, and Garrison. Only a few blocks away from the church where Finney sometimes preached was a Graham flour mill.[46] Through the practice of didactic exhortation, these men lectured and preached to the denizens of Rochester to replace predestination with the idea that humans could perfect themselves and their world (Finney); create a perfected way of life through abstention from the evils of meat, spices, and sex, especially "the solitary vice" (Graham); examine one's inner self to escape the conformities and achieve a change of heart (Emerson); or rid the nation of the sin of slavery (Garrison).[47]

Rochester also reveals how the embrace of these evangelisms had something to do with the struggle over status in a rapidly changing society. Fortune-seeking in America was a risky enterprise, and unstable economic conditions meant that "many men struggled from year to year, their economic state marginal and fluctuating."[48] Financial instability—particularly twenty years of antebellum boom and bust cycles—sent nearly a third of the American middle class careening between prosperity and insolvency.[49] Economic instability in places like Rochester—situated at the Western frontier of a rapidly transitioning American economy—made the free labor narrative of wage labor moving to small proprietorship more of a roller coaster between financial success and struggle. In this environment, stable respectability became more dependent on morality than property. Virtue, the moral righteousness that in the Revolutionary era was a mark of citizenship, became a form of class distinction. A purified lifestyle became a way for the middle classes to distinguish themselves from the working class, and self-righteous reform movements led the way to define and elevate this form of life. Therefore, the Northern Yankee culture of reform morality became a way to represent respectability for an emergent status-seeking urban Northern middle class.

Through this new and emerging group, reformers gained a powerful tool in the struggle for cultural prominence.[50] Yankee reformers could proclaim moral ideals that justified the prominence of older elites while providing a way for newcomers to fashion themselves as middle class.[51] A new, emerging professional class, not proprietors but clerks, professionals, and managers, who were gaining a foothold over and above the working class, could use the ideals of moral respectability to proclaim their new economic status as independent of owning property, a way of gaining social equality free of Jeffersonian definitions.

In establishing or joining these reform movements, Rochester's middle classes could also distinguish themselves from the newly arrived Irish and

German workers who came to build the Erie Canal in the 1820s. These new immigrant workers were disconnected from and not beholden to Anglo social strictures of small proprietorship, yeoman agriculture, the disappearing apprentice system, or traditional village paternalism.[52] The arrival of these new, nondeferential immigrant workers, along with economic upheavals such as the Panic of 1837, meant that the paternal older families and the emerging and insecure middle class both feared the laboring classes and feared becoming them. Within these anxious social conditions, those who survived financial busts intact "tended to conflate economic standing with moral virtue. Poverty was a personal failing, a secular sin."[53] By the 1840s, therefore, it is not surprising that Rochester's revivalists, along with their Boston cousins, formed the vanguard of active temperance, abolition, charitable, and "moral reform" societies, and, eventually, suffrage. It is no accident that Rochester was the home of Elizabeth Cady Stanton and Susan B. Anthony, and that Frederick Douglass moved there in the 1840s to start his newspaper, *The North Star*.

Nature

The English Romantic poet Percy Bysshe Shelley was, characteristically, both a vegetarian and a social reformer. He ended his 1813 pamphlet *A Vindication of Natural Diet* with the following block capital command: "NEVER TAKE ANY SUBSTANCE INTO THE STOMACH THAT ONCE HAD LIFE." Together, British and American Romanticism created "a structure of feeling and a set of rhetorical strategies employed by the emergent bourgeoisie to authorize and direct its political and economic ambitions."[54] The embrace of nature by British Romantics seeded and was seeded by the American Transcendentalists. The rejection of normal codes and an embrace of the natural went hand in hand on both sides of the Atlantic. Timothy Morton, describing Britain, states: "Vegetarianism was pervasive during the Romantic Period." Yet he also describes the philosophy behind this practice as "inconsistent": "it was both a means to rise above one's carnal animality and a way of returning to nature."[55] American utopian vegetarianism was similarly inconsistent in its philosophy. Like the British, American vegetarians sought to overcome their carnal desires for luxurious and "stimulating" foods. Yet they also looked to nature for the right way to live.

New scientific discoveries of the period also inspired reformers to look to universal laws of nature as a means to perfect one's lifestyle. Finney's self-made salvation pointed to a moral politics of personal life. Graham translated this moral politics into scientific choices about what to eat, making science a romantic quest in nature, to discover a perfect way of life in which "human life and health, and thought and feeling are governed by laws as precise and fixed and immutable as those which hold the planets in their orbits."[56] The immutable laws he found in nature all seemed to point toward abstemiousness, temperance, and self-control. Graham's ideas of self-improvement included all sorts of abstentions in addition to liquor: meat, fat, condiments, white bread, and too much sex, particularly of the solitary kind. While vilified by butchers and bakers, Graham lectured widely from Maine to Michigan throughout the 1830s. He described his proscribed foods as unnatural in that they overstimulated the appetite and thereby fostered lust, a lack of control.[57]

While Graham had retired from lecture touring and writing by the 1840s, followers of his precepts, mostly in the urban North, "crafted a Grahamite community through building and living in public institutions aimed at gaining converts and saving lost carnivores."[58] Followers lived in or ate in Grahamite boardinghouses in various Northeastern cities and read his writings in his books or the *Graham Journal of Health* or, later, the *Library of Health,* the journal of the American Physiological Society, founded by physician and fellow vegetarian reformer William Alcott. Followers also often visited associated "water cure" sanitariums, where fresh air and frequent washings were considered a cure for most illnesses. Whether in boardinghouses or sanatoriums, individuals believed that they "had a responsibility to regulate their own bodies by taking control over what they ingested," combining self-control with an embrace of nature.[59] In his writings on the cause of cholera, Graham blamed the "unnatural" consumption of meat and Americans who "were detached from and ignorant of the natural laws that regulated the human body, and drunk from a diet heavy in stimulants."[60] William Alcott, like Graham, wrote about the evils of overeating and advised avoiding rich and stimulating foods such as condiments and sugar.[61]

Europe

The lack of an aristocratic heritage meant that the emergent antebellum middle class were in want of a cultural foundation upon which to confirm their social status. Historian Lawrence Levine argues that the middle class sacralized not just evangelical vision but also Europe as a source of "high" culture:

"The process of sacralization reinforced the all too prevalent notion that for the source of divine inspiration and artistic creation one had to look not only upward but eastward toward Europe."[62] In their embrace of European culture, the antebellum North and South were in agreement. Yet, each section drew from different parts of European culture. While the South was increasingly enamored of the aristocratic ideals of honor, Northerners like Emerson were motivated by European Romanticism and its reaction against aristocratic culture. The Transcendentalists, for example, gained inspiration from the British Romantics like Coleridge and the German Idealists. American reformers therefore drew from British Romantics like Shelley and Byron, while European presses were the first to publish black abolitionist Phyllis Wheatley's poetry, making Romantic-era reform "a complex pattern of transatlantic exchange"[63] in which "the Atlantic was crossed and recrossed by reformers."[64]

Romantic reform was therefore a Northern, particularly Yankee, moral culture. Grahamite boardinghouses were popular primarily in Northern cities, and abstinence-based associations such as temperance organizations emerged primarily among the urban middle class in growing Northern cities. European Romantic reform, particularly for those not set on fire by evangelism, provided another path to middle-class cultural status, enabling Northerners to sacralize European culture while avoiding the taint of aristocracy. In doing so, they could also reject the European aristocratic notions of honor embraced as an alternative moral culture in the South.

REJECTING REFORM: SOUTHERN CULTURE

The foremost voice against abolition was, of course, the South. By the 1830s, Southerners had mostly rejected "organized political dissent, particularly dissent hostile to the expansion of slavery."[65] Along with this move came a rejection of the Yankee moral reform discourse that permeated the national, Northern print media. These newspapers and magazines increasingly equated the virtues of self-control with Northern ways of life and progressively isolated Southerners from public intellectual and moral discourse. While much of the intellectual strength of the Declaration of Independence and the Constitution had come from Southerners, by the Jacksonian era the South, even to many Southerners, had become an intellectual backwater. "Southern colleges," according to one observer, "were often institutions of higher learning only 'in name.'" Southern literary periodicals "seemed inevitably to fail; regional publishing facilities were inadequate," leaving the region, according to another observer, "defiled with ignorance."[66] Southern writers like Edgar Allen Poe struggled to create a Southern literary aristocracy and print culture that spoke to the American nation. Yet, attempts to create a national print culture emanating from the South failed due to both lack of printing facilities and lack of readers.[67]

Southerners also rejected the Northern moral culture of self-control and moderation, including abstinent ways of eating. While Southerners were not strong temperance reformers at any time in the nineteenth century, due in part to the economic need to move Southern corn crops in the transportable form of whiskey, the Southern temperance movements that did exist early in the nineteenth century were abandoned in the 1830s as these became increasingly associated with abolitionism.[68]

Yet, Southerners shared with Northern reformers the reaction against a materialist economic culture and "the kind of aggressive, mercenary, self-made man who was rapidly making his way in their society. In everyone's eyes this type of parvenu came to express a worrisome facet of the national character, to symbolize, in fact, both the restless mobility and the strident materialism of new world society."[69] However, unlike Northern reformers, Southerners reacted against this new type of American by embracing European aristocratic notions of chivalry, remaking the Northern notion of the slaveholder who shunned labor into the Cavalier, a role that emphasized dueling, generosity, hospitality, and notions of honor. These ideas were particularly inspired by the novels of Sir Walter Scott. In *Life on the Mississippi,* Mark Twain goes so far as to pin the cause of the Civil War on Scott's novels, particularly *Ivanhoe,* which tells of the gallant resistance of an honorable culture of Saxons against a tyrannical Norman overlord. Southerners read Scott's novel as an allegory for their own condition, and proclaimed themselves as a separate Saxon culture, apart from the moral tenets of Yankee Northerners. Scott "had so large a hand in making Southern character, as it existed before the war," Twain wrote, that Scott was not only "responsible for the war," but also, after the war, for something he calls "Sir Walter Scott disease," which trapped the South in a static culture.

Yet, in the 1830s and '40s, many in both the North and South looked to the Southern gentleman as the source of an antimaterialist way of life. Like the abolitionist reformers and the Transcendentalists, many Northerners saw the rise of a new grasping, avaricious merchant class as threatening democratic society, and some looked to the "legendary Southern gentleman" as an alternative culture. The Southern gentleman "seemed to possess every quality that the Yankee lacked: honor and integrity, indifference to money and business, a decorous concern for the amenities, and a high sense of civic and social responsibility."[70] Sarah Josepha Hale, for example, in her novels and other writings, presented the South as "less a place than a moral climate: an expression of what the North lacked and what the emergent Yankee needed."[71] The ideal, for Hale, was a combination of Northern and Southern traits: a gentleman who was disinterested in money-making and dedicated to social and civil society while being self-controlled and self-disciplined in his personal life. While abolitionists adapted the early nineteenth-century concern about the American character and self-improvement to an abstemious way of life, the public audience tended to prefer Hale's vision of American character that was a synthesis between Northern and Southern ideas of a life beyond materialist greed. The idea of abstemious self-denial as virtue also contradicted the role of magazine print culture dependent on advertising. Southern virtues fit more neatly into the emerging consumer culture.

For the South, the Southern gentleman—the Cavalier—was a mythical being who represented a more reflective way of life less interested in money than in "the genial elegancies of social life."[72] The Southern rejection of Northern reform movements was therefore not based on slaveholding alone; instead, it was a broader struggle over ways of life, and that way of life included food. Meat-eating, luxurious diets, and rich comfort foods therefore became a form of resistance to the moral authority of Yankee reformers. Southern culture provided an alternative code of antebellum gentility that was attractive to the emerging middle class who wanted to enjoy the comforts of their new wealth. Northern reformers repulsed by Southern slaveholding therefore had to wage a battle for the hearts of the general public attracted by the shared culture of comfort and well-being de Tocqueville identified in *Democracy in America.*

Food became one arena in which Northern reformers and the slaveholding South were locked in battle to define American morality. Prized by Southern women, "[t]he groaning table of southern cuisine, heavily laden with baked, stewed, creamed and beaten burdens, attests in cookbook, memoir, and fiction to the hospitality of the southern home."[73] Hospitality revolved around providing large quantities of rich food, the very kind of "luxurious eating" Northern reformers warned against.[74] And hospitality required that this food be available on a daily basis to any friends and visitors who might "drop in": antebellum Southern cookbooks describe the ideal household as one in which the husband can invite a friend to dinner "in full confidence of finding his wife unruffled . . . who can usher his guest into the dining-room assured of seeing that methodical nicety which is the essence of true elegance."[75]

From the opposite pole, Northern women, particularly abolitionist writers like Catharine Beecher, also defined food as central to the politics of slavery, but made their focus not the dining room but the kitchen. Her sister, Harriet Beecher Stowe, set much of *Uncle Tom's Cabin* in the slave kitchen.[76] In choosing the kitchen as the center of the home, Beecher was following the notions of virtue as described in Northern middle-class literature of the time, which "featured the kitchen as the heart of the household." Comparing Northern and Southern literature of the time, Evelyn Fox Genovese argues that Northern women reformers defined the kitchen as the romantic place of a refined and civilized life where "housework became nurture and the woman's prescribed toil became a mission of love." Southern women, in contrast, "shared a distaste for housework and an uneasy relation to the bourgeois and evangelical virtues of work, thrift and cleanliness." In Southern plantation homes, the kitchen was "honored" by "expelling it from the house."[77]

Southern women like Mary Chestnut rejected the Northern sacralization of the kitchen as "piety & . . . pie . . . . Such baking and brewing—the house maid's duties elevated to the highest scale of human refinement."[78] Yet, Southerners defined themselves by the food they—that is, their slaves—provided. Hospitality—the giving of pleasure to one's guests through the provision of entertainment and pleasure—remained at the center of Southern culture. Southern antebellum literature from the period is full of plantation owners gone bankrupt due to their expenditures entertaining guests. One novel describes how a bankrupt planter goes into hiding to avoid entertainment expenditures that would put him into deeper debt. But rather than being a cautionary tale, this narrative is seen as part of the definition of Southern honor. The Southern gentleman was self-indulgent and indulgent of others, "men who, so long as they could command the means, by sale of their last acre, or last negro, would have a good dinner, and give a hearty welcome to whomsoever chose to drop in, to eat, friend or stranger, bidden or unbidden."[79] From the perspective of Southern hospitality, self-denial and disciplined eating was a kind of uncivil parsimony, a kind of selfishness.[80]

The division between Northern middle-class reformers and Northern wageworkers in some ways paralleled the division between Northerners and

Southerners. Reform groups during this time period sought, through lectures, newspapers, and the distribution of tracts, to evangelize workers to convert to an abstemious way of life. Moral suasion to change hearts against slavery was also moral suasion to change workers' hearts against moral habits that reformers saw as the source of workers' misery and a support of slave culture.[81] Yet, despite the urgings of the reformers, workers, like Southerners, sought comfort and indulgence rather than self-control. And those defending the South and slavery understood their shared interests with Northern workers. Slavery's apologists in the South seized upon the inability of Northern reformers to see the role of social inequality in the creation of working-class exploitation. Numerous Southern authors used working-class inequality as a reason for the superiority of the slave system, based on the idea that free labor was free to starve while slaveowners "cared" for their labor. As a result "[s]everal trade unionists in the antebellum North agreed with slavery's apologists that not only the working and living conditions but in some respects the 'liberty' enjoyed by Northern hirelings compared unfavorably with the situation of slaves."[82] Northerners, on the other hand, were "united by a commitment to a 'free labor ideology,' grounded in the precepts that free labor was economically and socially superior to slave labor and that the distinctive quality of Northern society was the opportunity it offered wage earners to rise to property-owning independence" but only through self-control and hard work.[83]

These sectional and class disagreements were reflected in party politics. In the early 1800s, the antislavery Whig Party "appealed to middle- and upper-class folk in relatively prosperous rural areas, towns, and cities" both North and South, as well as "to some portions of the urban working class."[84] Whigs tended to be the older, more patrician American families and more professional workers in both regions. Yet, by the 1840s, a stronger, more political form of antislavery emerged, in response to the Fugitive Slave Law, which forced Northerners to catch and return escaped slaves. Questions of the status of slavery in newly settled states in the West, as well as incidents where Northerners directly experienced the arrest and return of escaped slaves, brought the slavery question directly into the Whig and emergent Republican parties, the latter of which became a party of the North. In contrast, Jacksonian Democrats, North and South, combined to embrace a less-government, less-interference platform that included not interfering with either private life or in slave states. The Democratic Party in the North also tended to represent newer immigrant groups who were often Catholic, while Whigs—and Whig reformers—were older Protestant families concerned about the protection of the traditional republican virtues of piety and self-control.[85]

PURIFIED UTOPIAS

The more radical of the Northern reformers viewed these tensions as the struggle between purity and corruption. Freeing the country from slavery meant purifying it. Yet, Rush's emphasis on balance and temperance became, in the hands of radical reformers, a hyper-purification process by which people solved problems through repurifying, building stronger boundaries between purity and corruption, resulting in a continual struggle to remove all evidence of corruption in life practices. One example of this purification treadmill was the attempt to establish morally perfect places, utopian communities, throughout upstate New York and the wider Northeastern region. In these communities, reformers developed purified ways of life and then set out to live from these—often abstract—precepts. Brook Farm was a relatively tolerant Transcendentalist community that included more omnivorous intellectuals like Emerson and Thoreau as consistent guests. Yet even at Brook Farm there was a special table at dinner for the Grahamites. Brook Farm member and fervent abolitionist and education reformer Bronson Alcott, cousin of William Alcott and father of Louisa May, believed that Brook Farm did not go far enough in creating a new way of life that would accomplish the "change of heart" necessary to purify American society. In 1843, in partnership with British Romantic evangelist Charles Lane, Alcott established a new community along perfectionist lines: Fruitlands.

In the communal living experiment at Fruitlands, utopia depended on the highly disciplined behavior of the participants, which centered on vegetarianism. This radical community went far to overturn generally accepted rules of public behavior while subjecting members to strict discipline. Alcott was a friend of Emerson's, and his description of the "seekers" describes Fruitlands' inhabitants and their precepts remarkably well. These utopians not only rejected meat, but also abjured the use of animals because plowing and manuring were a "debauchery of both the earthly soil and of the human body."[86] At Fruitlands, as Emerson described it, "the farm must be spaded." Abjurance and abstinence were Fruitlands' major rules, and anyone who violated these rules was expelled. Concern about the corruption of product made by slaves or from animals meant that members wore linen clothes and canvas shoes. "The entrance to paradise is still through the strait and narrow gate of self-denial," wrote Alcott.

By purifying their lives, rejecting all that was associated with the evils of the world—not just the slave-grown sugar or the colonial coffee and tea, but any ingestion of foods that required using another being as property—these reformers believed they could provide a new model to the world of the right way to live. This way of life, evangelized by Alcott and Lane through the lecture circuit, would catch on because it was perfect and pure. Their didactic exhortations were more inspired by the European Romantic mystics, such as Swedenborg, and the European socialists than by Finney's evangelism. These mystical ideas, which also influenced Emerson, took the universe as a source of wisdom that could inspire new forms of human organization. When perfected, these new ways of life would purify the world into an Eden where even climate and the solar system would transform into a perfect unity with human life.[87]

Fruitlands residents exemplified the apostles described by Emerson: the small group lived an abstinent life, while Alcott and Lane spent much of their time away from the community, evangelizing the lifestyle epitomized there. Their didactic exhortations included a night at Emerson's home where, according to Emerson's notes, they came to "unfold as far as they can their idea of a true social institution."[88] For Alcott and Lane, the moral culture based on private property was as sinful as meat. This rejection of private property stemmed both from socialist ideas and from Alcott's strong abolitionist beliefs: a refusal to participate in a world tainted with humans as property widened into a rejection of all forms of property ownership, including animals.

But Alcott's community, described in ironic detail by his daughter, Louisa May, in her essay "Transcendental Wild Oats," comprised less than a dozen participants. Despite its lofty goals, many of the stories that have come out of this experience are about food, showing the links between social reform and dietary reform. Louisa May Alcott described how one resident was banished for eating fish.[89] Another young man, Isaac Hecker, wrote in his diary about how his two-week experience at Fruitlands confirmed his commitment to live on bread, fruit, and nuts. In his twenties at the time, he suffered from multiple gastric, angelic, and romantic visitations that a simple diet seemed to relieve.[90] He later went on to found the Paulist Fathers, a Catholic evangelical sect devoted to converting all of the United States to Catholicism.

In those long decades before Emancipation, abolitionists worked to end slavery and were frustrated by their inability to foment change. While these reformers were clearly in the right about slavery, it is worth considering whether their social reform through self-reform and conversion to a particular set of morals was an effective tool to end this injustice. Freedom for slaves did not eventually come about through moral suasion or the purification of personal lives, but rather through cumulative political crises and a violent civil war.

Romantic reformers, on the other hand, have had an immense impact on the strategies of subsequent American reform movements. "Despite the failure of moral suasion to end slavery," states historian T. Gregory Garvey, "Garrison was the single most important figure in creating the institutional structure of the culture of reform. In the connection he emphasized between the moral character of the individual and the authority to make political demands in the secular public sphere, Garrison integrated the ideal of republican virtue with self-purifying Evangelical conversion into a single model of democratic citizenship."[91] Perfectionist civic romanticism—the search for the perfect alternative—became the way to solve American problems, the national ideal of the democratic citizen. Yet, the inadequacy of personal purification to solve social problems meant that Perfectionist reformers became caught in a treadmill of purity in which failure to change society through personal change led to greater personal purification and repurification to the point of debilitation. Fruitlands represents the apex of this strategy for social reform.

American social movements have continued to share this ideology of personal purification as the road to social change, a romantic search for the pure life and a rejection of current society as corrupt. Like the abolitionists' romantic envisioning of a perfect new world beyond the human bondage of slavery, American reform movements have been hampered by their inability to see issues beyond the dichotomies of good and bad, of solving social problems through personal virtue that purifies a corrupt world. This approach leaves reformers blind to the struggle between classes, political parties, and sections of the country. In a world where social change is a struggle between fixed imaginaries, realist paths to a better future disappear. Rather than breaking down this boundary, reformers cross and recross the boundary, reclaiming either a perfect inside or a perfect outside of society as the solution to social problems.

Freeing the country from slavery did not result from a moral crusade of purification but through a messy political fight and bloody national conflict.

Yet, the glorification of abolitionists for their clearly correct moral stand—or the continued vilification of the abolitionists by "Lost Cause" Southerners—has hidden the fact that the processes that ended slavery had little or nothing to do with personal purification or "change of heart." The history of antislavery politics shows that contests over slavery were fought not only in churches and reform associations but also in a political arena that addressed the broader struggle over ideas of freedom and order. But moral reformers' rejection of politics in favor of purification belied the commonalities of ideology between abolitionists and antislavery politicians. As a result, industrial interests co-opted reform agendas after the war, focusing on reformers' personal discipline agenda instead of larger struggles for freedom by newly emancipated blacks and industrial workers, both of whom became targets for reform moralizing.

Food historians have noted the link between abolition and vegetarianism.[92] This chapter showed us why. The chapters in Part II will show how abolitionism, despite its "apartness" from its own time, became the blueprint for American reform movements, "shap[ing] public discourse in ways that *still* define the manner in which Americans deal with divisive issues."[93] For this reason, in anticipation of Part II it is important to explore the link between Romantic reform movements' focus on dietary purification as a central strategy. As Part II will subsequently demonstrate, it is this Romantic reform fervor that pervades the food reform movements of today.

3

Gut Wars

GILDED AGE STRUGGLES AGAINST PURITY

THE MILITARY VICTORY of the Northern states ended the struggle between the moral ideals of the North and the South. Northern Yankee moral culture, combining ideals of the self-controlled virtuous citizen with the ideal of the free labor self-made man, became the national culture of democratic citizenship in an orthocratic order of moral purity. This nationalizing of Yankee moral culture, however, was transformed by the industrial juggernaut wakened by the Civil War—and increasingly presided over by the new faith in science—overcoming the Transcendentalist rejection of materialism. What was previously seen as Yankee acquisitiveness and selfishness became the pure, superior, and triumphant culture of efficiency, thrift, and productivity. Reformers embraced what they shared with industrialists: ideals about order and freedom through discipline and hard work. In tandem, reformers began to evolve into the professional class, entering, and sometimes establishing, the emerging institutions of health, sanitation, food, and nutrition.

The Yankee moral culture of free labor, efficiency, productivity, and self-control became the ideal cultural citizenship of a newly unified and reordered nation. Along with this moral ideal came an ideal diet. At the forefront of the development of national institutions of public health and nutrition, New England reformers made the Yankee diet the ideal form of American eating. The triumph of Yankee moral culture as the definition of the national ideal, however, meant that some Americans were excluded in the definition of ideal citizens and stigmatized as disorderly. These groups included newly freed African Americans, who struggled for the right to land to achieve subsistence; recalcitrant Southerners of the "Problem South," who shared a regional comfort cuisine with African Americans; and foreigners like the Chinese, who ate less meat. In turn, Northern white workers used this new national moral culture as a way to claim superiority in the workplace and as rightful citizens.

The moral precepts of the self-controlled citizen developed by the American Founders was transformed into moral reform movements aimed at creating a disciplined workforce of self-controlled producers and eaters.[1] The Yankee morality of self-control joined with economic notions of efficiency through scientific analysis of worker efficiency. A new middle class of scientific professionals emerged out of Yankee reform culture, with a new didactic task: to transform producers—workers and farmers—into a more efficient and productive machine by teaching them discipline and thrift through scientific ideas about health and diet. Northern moral culture came to define the national moral—and dietary—ideal in terms of rational productivity and efficiency.

Yet, the Southern definition of American freedom as equality and pleasure did not disappear. The new, emerging commercial culture took up the idea of pleasure and comfort as a legitimate aspect of American life, worthy of pursuit by all. Increasingly, the tension between self-control and pleasure was played out between American commercial culture, which promised pleasures and comforts, and reformer-professionals who exhorted citizens to maintain discipline and self-control. Workers resisting reformers' didactic exhortations could find solace in the comforts and pleasures promised by the new commercial culture. New products and inventions promised to resolve the tensions between self-discipline and comfort by giving purchasers the ability to experience pleasure without consequence.

Dietary conversations in the Reconstruction Era set the stage for the move to industrial efficiency as both workplace discipline and the promise of comfort through the provision of cheap luxuries for the working class. In turn, the culture of civic reform evolved into the culture of expertise, as didactic culture moved into the emerging industrial, government, and university institutions, as well as the expanding print culture. Most histories of work efficiency start with Frederick Winslow Taylor and the time studies of workers in the 1880s and 1890s.[2] Yet, *The American Woman's Home,* Catharine Beecher's and Harriet Beecher Stowe's widely read book that was first published in 1869, provides an analysis of working efficiency in the kitchen that predated Taylor's work on the factory floor. Beecher and Stowe were at the forefront of women seeking to make housekeeping—particularly cooking—expert, efficient, and clean, precursors to the work that later became the profession of home economics.

The idea of efficient diets did not go uncontested. Workers did not forget what they were working for: prosperity and comfort, not self-denial. Workers therefore resisted attempts to transform them into more thrifty dietary consumers. Once again, the struggle was over meat, with workers standing by their perceived right to eat more meat than other workers around the world. The working class voiced many of its demands for higher wages in terms of the equal right to share in America's dietary riches—and richness. Struggles over wages often became struggles over meat-eating. Reformers, therefore, rather than advocating vegetarianism, worked to create more efficient diets with moderate amounts of inexpensive meat.

Reformers' efforts to make workers more thrifty in their eating habits received strong industry support, since thrifty eating meant less pressure to raise wages. But, the commercial culture's promise of comfort, pleasure, and prosperity bloomed with the new industrial economy. The wealthy girth became a display of this prosperous promise, as "fat cats" celebrated their success with lavish meals. Southerners also continued to eat, and to celebrate, their regional dietary habits, and their comforting and rich meals became a kind of resistance to the Northern culture of self-denial. Rich Southern food was a signpost of what a "rich" life could be: tempting, indulgent, aristocratic, celebratory, and comforting.

Advertisers embraced this other side of American culture, making consumer culture the tempting antidote to the orthocratic moral order. Advertisements emphasized the ability to seek pleasure, to "eat what I please" without bodily punishment. In this struggle, freedom as control was countered by a different notion: freedom from control, especially the control of dietary advice. Advertisers played into this desire with products that linked comfort with health, as in patent medicines that promised "eat all you want" and by portraying rich and flavorful products as temptations that brought happiness (fig. 3). Consumer products, such as laxatives, promoted new technologies as a way to resolve the contradictions inherent in this high-consumption way of life. These products drew on ideas of American freedom, as they seized the opportunity to make a profit by seemingly resolving the struggle between "eating what I want" and "eating what I should." Commercial products beckoned as solutions to this dilemma, promising new ingestive freedoms. To be able to eat what you want, without consequences, was advertising's new vision of freedom and led to the growth in sales of patent-medicine stomach remedies, laxatives, and diet pills.

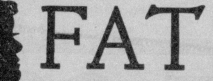
FIGURE 3. Late nineteenth-century advertisements for popular weight-loss patent medicines.

The following examples show that struggles over diet reflected larger Gilded Age struggles. It begins with a story of the dietary struggles between emancipated slaves and Northern industrialists, mediated through abolitionist reformers. In the vanquished South, the regional diet became a sign of degeneracy rather than comfort, as the Northern dairy-intensive diet became increasingly defined as national food practice. Struggles between industrialists and their Northern urban workers also played out in dietary advice, mediated by Northern reformers. Finally, workers' struggle over wages became a struggle between different working-class ethnic groups, linking the reform idea of one national dietary culture and the stigmatization of other regional and ethnic diets. These conflicts remained within, but redefined, the American notion of comfort and order, as a new group of professional nutritionists emerged to negotiate these tensions through science.

THE AGROECOLOGY OF EMANCIPATION: "NO MORE PECK OF CORN"

The first arena for this emerging struggle was in the Northern-occupied section of the slave states during the Civil War. The diet of slaves varied by place, plantation, regional culture, and whim of the plantation owner. However, black freedmen serving as soldiers in the Civil War sang as a group, "No more peck of corn for me," while they marched, recognizing the most common ration for slaves.[3] Corn was the major staple food in the South, for black and white, both before and after Emancipation, with some fatback or hog meat commonly added to this ration.[4] Yet, some slaves grew gardens and raised chickens, sometimes for sale and sometimes for their own consumption.[5]

Struggles over diet in the Northern-occupied South began as a tension over what to grow—that is, what would be the new system of land and labor. Answers to this question began with new growing-system experiments that began during the Civil War, in the Sea Islands and Low Country of South Carolina and Georgia, areas emancipated only a few months after the conflict began. Here, the struggle can be described as agroecological, a term currently used to describe today's sustainable food systems. However, a more general definition of agroecology is the relationship between society, nature, and economy. The agroecological question after Emancipation became therefore: What new system of growing would emerge out of a vanquished plantation system and a newly freed labor force?

The Sea Islands were a good place to start formulating this agroecological alternative. The slave culture in these islands was more autonomous, due to the islands' isolation and the prevalence of malaria, which meant that owners left slaves to themselves for large parts of the year. Here, slave work was organized according to the "task" system, in which slave cultivators were assigned a certain amount of work each day, with the rest of the day available for growing their own subsistence crops such as vegetables or poultry.[6] The transformation of this system during the war and after Emancipation involved the struggle over land that was also a struggle over diet, in this case between newly freed slaves and those who were looking for a new system of labor for growing cotton for Northern factories.

Because of their vulnerability to naval attack, the Sea Islands were taken by Union troops only seven months after Fort Sumter, and it was here that abolitionist General Rufus Saxton decided to show "the capabilities of the Negro for freedom and self-support and self-improvement, to determine whether he is specifically distinct from and inferior to the white race, and normally a slave or dependent, or only inferior by accident of position and circumstances, still a man, and entitled to all the rights which our organic law has declared belongs to all men by the endowment of the Creator."[7] Saxton was put in command of the "Port Royal Experiment," a test of whether slaves, once freed, could fulfill Northern Yankee moral ideals of the good American citizen.

Despite the unique culture of the Sea Islands slave communities, the struggles over the definition of freedom and order as it applied to these communities represented, in microcosm, the struggles over the nature of freedom and order for the emancipated slave in the South as a whole. The slaves quickly transformed the cotton plantations into subsistence agricultural communities, growing vegetables, sweet potatoes, and corn. Figure 4 is a photograph of "James Hopkinson's Plantation," on Edisto Island, where freed slaves were planting crops for their own subsistence. Hopkinson did not reclaim the land until 1866.[8] In the absence of owners, slaves claimed plots for themselves and began to set themselves up as smallholders. Saxton granted titles to some of the plantation land.

With the arrival of Union troops in the Sea Islands came a group of abolitionist missionaries, known as "Gideon's Band," intent on setting up schools and other forms of "improvement" for the new freedmen. The missionaries were sent to teach reading but, more importantly, "the mutual restraints and civilities of social order."[9] Along with the missionaries came representatives

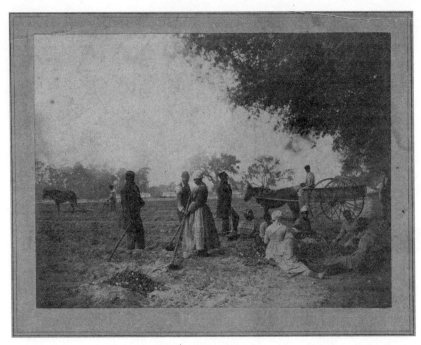

FIGURE 4. Henry P. Moore, "Sweet Potatoe Planting—James Hopkinson's Plantation," Edisto Island, South Carolina, April 8, 1862. Photographs and Prints Division. Schomburg Center for Research in Black Culture, New York Public Library, Astor, Lenox and Tilden Foundations.

of Northern industrialists, who exhorted the slaves to plant the high-quality, long-staple cotton of Sea Islands plantation agriculture. The freedmen accepted the offer of education but initially refused to grow cotton. They had already destroyed or hidden the cotton gins, vowing never to participate in that agricultural system again. Instead, they preferred to maintain their small acreage in the cultivation of crops that composed their diet, what they had grown as "provisions" in the plantation system.[10] Not needing the income from cotton, freed slaves could not see any reason to grow it, and "like the farm workers of the North, they became ambitious to work for themselves, to own farms of their own."[11] In the cotton system, most land went to the production of a market crop; without cotton, there was plenty of land to feed the newly freed inhabitants. Slaves in many areas, but especially in the Low Country, had long participated in the local market system, raising livestock and other foods for sale to whites and each other.[12] In the Sea Islands' agroecological system, where slaves had traditionally provided for themselves, why grow cotton if you didn't have to support the plantation owner?

Republicans were divided about how to handle Southern lands after the Civil War, but they all agreed that free labor, the right to sell one's labor for wages, was "the central meaning of Reconstruction: the replacement of an unfair, morally destructive, unproductive system with the purportedly democratic, intrinsically fair, and efficient system of wage labor."[13] Abolitionists were so tied to the free labor ideology that they believed "labor and capital shared the same basic interests, and second, that employers and employees were equal parties to the construction of contracts."[14] Yet, the idea of subsistence and local market agriculture replacing cotton agriculture in the South conflicted with the interests of Northern textile industrialists and with the free labor ideology of the abolitionists and the Republican Party. Edward Philbrick, one of the Port Royal reformers who was also an industrialist, noted, "the abandonment of slavery did not imply the abandonment of cotton."[15] Massachusetts Emancipation Society member Edward Atkinson, the same textile industrialist who had helped to finance John Brown's Harpers Ferry raid, worked closely with Philbrick and the Port Royal Northerners, involved first with the military occupation administration in the Sea Islands and later with the Freedmen's Bureau, to reorganize cotton production. Before the war, Atkinson had argued that free men could grow cotton more efficiently. Atkinson's opinion was immensely influential in Washington, representing industrial interests. Mark Twain said of him in *Life on the Mississippi*: "an opinion from Mr. Edward Atkinson upon any vast national commercial matter, comes as near ranking as authority, as can the opinion of any individual in the Union."[16]

Responding to these pressures, Union officials worked to convince the freedmen to work for wages in the cotton fields. Saxton called "the Port Royal Experiment" successful: freedmen "demonstrated at least as much willingness to work for wages as white Americans."[17] When General Sherman's Field Order #15 allotted refugees and Sea Islanders forty-acre homesteads, ex-slaves even more clearly saw themselves as practicing the ideology of autonomy and self-sufficiency through property ownership that had been part of the Founders' conversation: "More land was cultivated than ever before, and cotton fields were kept in excellent shape. Plenty of corn, tomatoes, okra, melons and potatoes were planted. Chickens and vegetables were sold in the Charleston market to bring farmers needed cash. Not only did the people dress and eat better than ever in their lives; they now worked only six or seven hours a day."[18]

Yet, the promise of land titles by the Freedmen's Bureau—and actually given to Sea Islands farmers—was eventually voided. Much of the land was auctioned off to Northern speculators, many of them from antislavery and abolitionist families.[19] The "New Masters" from the North included Philbrick himself, who reconstituted the system of plantation labor for growing cotton based on paying wage labor to now landless freedmen. While the long-staple cotton of the Sea Islands was not used in Northern factories, Northern industrialists considered the Port Royal Experiment a testing ground for rebuilding cotton production in other areas. As the "occupied Confederacy" expanded with Northern victories, particularly in Mississippi, Northern businessmen, many associated with antislavery groups that had restructured finance to re-equip Southern plantations for production, bought leases. While welcoming emancipated labor, Northern financiers of New York and Boston "feared that the newly emancipated black voters would fall under the control of dema-gogues who would call for the punishment of whites and for confiscation and redistribution of white-owned lands." Northern industrialist Edward Atkinson led in the restructuring of Southern cotton growing. Having argued before the war that cotton production would be more productive with free labor, he created financial institutions to effect this change. However, for Atkinson, free labor did not mean black ownership. Instead, he advocated organizing labor through contracts with white owners, which eventually became the sharecropping system of the cotton South. This abolitionist, now a representative of the Massachusetts Reconstruction Association, called the redistribution of land titles to freed blacks on former plantations in the Sea Islands "schemes of confiscation."[20] If blacks owned land, he and other indus-trialists feared, they would not grow enough cotton.[21]

In other words, abolitionists were heavily involved in the establishment of the sharecropping system. Abolitionist William Henry Brisbane was appointed Tax Commissioner for South Carolina and in charge of auction-ing off the properties at many times the price per acre of Homestead land—in conflict with Saxton. Saxton had argued that "[t]he immediate possession of the land without purchase is the indefeasible right of the negro" and had given and / or sold land title to a number of freedmen.[22] Those titles were mostly voided. While some, like Saxton, favored redistribution or sale in a Homestead Act type system, in fact, much of this land was auctioned off into the hands of Northerners.

Harriet Beecher herself bought a plantation in the South, primarily as a way to revive the mental health of her alcoholic son, but also to do the kind of missionary work there that she recommends in *The American Woman's Home:* to civilize a community in a state, Florida, that was then still a frontier. Living there each winter, she combined business interests with moral education, seeking to hire on labor contracts the newly freed slaves who came to settle there, while forming a school to train former female slaves to do housework.[23] Stowe's missionary work involved more than just training former slaves. She aspired to bring the Yankee "Christian Home" precepts to the South by creating an efficient and moral workforce, "well-trained servants—who could respect their positions and take pride in service,"[24] the kinds of servants being trained in the Northern cooking schools. However, she was quickly "used up and exhausted with the strain" of trying to teach her own servant, Minnah, how to keep house according to her book. Minnah, who had previously been a field hand, kept leaving the house to take care of her own animals, finally leaving permanently, shouting, "I don't want none o' your housework."[25]

As the sharecropping system developed and expanded, the practice of growing provisions for personal consumption was crowded out by the need to grow cotton: "The usual pattern was for croppers to work as much land in cotton as possible—often right up to the back door of their cabins—leaving little room for gardens." As a result, fresh vegetables "were probably a more common part of the Negro diet before 1860 than in the early 1940s." This explains much of the rise of Southern dietary diseases like pellagra, a disease that, ironically, later became another target of Northern nutritionist dietary reform.[26]

In other words, once the emancipated slaves joined the ranks of "free labor," abolitionists expected them to take on Yankee moral culture and also to participate in the commercial economy, the two major tenets of the free labor creed. Echoing the free labor narrative of wage labor leading to proprietorship, Freedmen's Bureau commissioner General Oliver Otis Howard envisioned a system where blacks "return to plantation labor, but under conditions that allowed them the opportunity to work their way out of the wage-earning class." He advised a black audience: "You must begin at the bottom of the ladder and climb up."[27] In the end, much of the land was auctioned off or returned to plantation owners.

In the decades following these events, the ravages of the boll weevil in Sea Islands cotton made agriculture less valuable and much of the land eventually reverted to black ownership, becoming the communities of Gullah culture. Freedmen in other parts of the South were not as fortunate. Some did buy land, but with the end of Reconstruction, left to their own devices and without even the promises of landownership that the Homestead Act provided to white settlers, most became sharecroppers throughout the South. By the turn of the century, abolitionists like Atkinson were writing editorials advocating immigration of free labor from Europe to settle Western lands to grow cotton and wheat. The idea of giving those who grew cotton in the South access to Western cotton lands was not considered. From the Northern reformers' point of view, freedmen's resistance to growing cotton proved that they were incapable of becoming Yankee proprietors.

Fifty years later, Zora Neale Hurston wrote *Their Eyes Were Watching God,* a novel set in the black South of the early twentieth century. In the book, food becomes a metaphor for freedom, the truly lived life: the protagonist, a young black woman, Janie Mae Crawford, escapes from a confining and loveless marriage through her love of the food-named "Tea Cake," a man who takes her to the bean-growing fields of Florida. Good food becomes a metaphor for the good life and a complete self, reminiscent of the dietary struggles post-emancipation, struggles that, for African Americans, were imbued with the desire for identity, diet, and the means to produce it, a dream of ingestive subjectivity, of physical and moral intactness.[28]

These historical and fictional narratives present the struggles of those outside of the boundaries of purity and order defined by Yankee culture. The abolitionist divided the world into virtuous citizens deemed capable of choice and control, of being the ideal American striving for autonomy through free labor, and those on the disorderly outside who were deemed incapable of autonomy. The definition of Yankee ingestive subjectivity as pure and orderly denied the moral intactness of those who chose to order their lives differently. As a result, "[s]tories of African American life often reflect the experiences of black people struggling to be full human beings in spite of the legacy of slavery and Jim Crow."[29] While the Yankee moral order triumphed as the national ideal, as the intact national political body composed of the intact bodies of its deserving citizens, those outside this ideal were politically dismembered, deemed incapable of self-control and orderly citizenship.

It is ironic that those most concerned about the freedom of slaves were those who carried out the Port Royal Experiments and who, in the end, declared the freed slaves undeserving of freedom. While some abolitionists, like Saxon, contended that the freedmen had passed the test, had shown their ability to be virtuous like their Yankee examiners, once the freed slaves were forced to meet the norms of Yankee virtue, they had already lost. By judging others according to their own ideals of purity and virtue, the Port Royal abolitionists denied the freed slaves their own cultural self-determination. The choice was either to give up their own selves and identities or to be declared undeserving. The Port Royal test presaged the end of Reconstruction, when white Southerners reclaimed political power and denied the rights of citizenship to African Americans by declaring them incapable of order. In sum, Port Royal represents the other side of the purity project: the dismembering of the bodily and cultural integrity of those marginalized by those bounded ideals.

STIGMATIZING SOUTHERN FOOD

The Civil War defeat enforced the notion of the South as degenerate in its ways of life and the North as exemplifying truly American moral ways of living. Beyond the Sea Islands, abolitionists looked to the conquered South as a place of mission. In *The American Woman's Home,* Beecher and Stowe describe the "destitute settlements" which "abound all over the West and South" and recommend that a "Christian family" settle in these places, which would cause "the desert to blossom as the rose."[30] Beecher even proposed a set of agricultural institutes, one in each Southern state, run by women.[31] Harriet Beecher Stowe's Florida plantation was meant to fulfill the missionary ideal of bringing Yankee culture to the South.

The South no longer held its place as part of the balancing of American culture against the onslaught of materialism. Northerner Albion Tourgée, transplanted to the South, echoed Northern sentiments when he described the region as a "magnificent failure." In Tourgée's novel, *A Fool's Errand,* the main character describes North and South as "convenient names for two distinct, hostile and irreconcilable ideas. . . . At the North . . . we are apt to speak of the one as civilization, and of the other as a species of barbarism."[32] Yankees, triumphant in war, evangelized not just Christianity across the South but also "never doubted that they were true pioneers of free labor, evangelists of a more excellent way."[33] Catherine Beecher exhorted Northeastern women to proselytize the gospel of virtuous living throughout the West and South. Her brother, preacher and missionary society leader Henry Ward Beecher, proclaimed that the country would be led by "northern men, with northern ideas, and with a northern gospel."[34]

Northern reformers took up their mission, proselytizing the right way to live and eat to the rest of the country. The 1870s witnessed the rise of cooking schools in the North, including the Boston Cooking School—later directed by Fannie Farmer—and Juliet Corson's New York Cooking School. Textbooks for these schools tended to emphasize Europeanized Yankee cooking. Corson's 1879 *Cooking School Text Book and Housekeepers' Guide to Cookery and Kitchen Management* is typical. It lists mostly European names for its mostly Yankified recipes, including such dishes as "Broiled *Filets* with *Maitre d'Hotel* butter" and "White *Haricot* Beans, *Bordelaise* Style." European cuisine from the cooking schools was not the Mediterranean cookery of olive oil and vegetables but the Northern European and Northern American diet emphasizing butter, milk, and, especially, cream sauces.[35] Increasingly challenged by competition from the frontier agriculture of corn and grain, the Northeast had moved more deeply into dairy production as the region's main agricultural economy, an agroecology that fit in well with the Northern European diet.[36] The Northeastern cooking schools sacralized this dairy-centered diet through the immersion of most foods in white sauce, a mixture of butter, flour, and milk or cream.[37] "This fondness for whitening their food before eating it became a habit," food historian Laura Shapiro notes. "Creamy sauces and garnishes were prescribed consistently in the menus" of the Boston and New York Cooking Schools, "so that soups arrived with whipped cream atop each bowl, tossed salads were smeared with boiled dressing or with mayonnaise mixed with whipped cream, and ice creams and Bavarian creams turned up for dessert covered with more cream."[38]

CLASS GUT WARS

While calories, fats, and proteins were inadequate in many diets around the nineteenth-century world, America was a haven for those seeking enough to eat. Immigrants, semi-starved in their own countries, arrived to America "hungry and in part because of hunger. America had achieved a deserved global reputation as a place where food could be had for relatively little money." The American dream for these immigrants was not the road paved with gold but with "tables sagging with food unimaginable to them back home." "The American workers . . . ate precisely those items which in Europe were defined as luxuries, food reserved for the upper classes, with meat and white flour bread high on the list."[39] By the time these immigrants had arrived, Americans "were eating meat on a scale that the Old World could neither imagine nor provide."[40] European workers, native and immigrant, therefore saw rich food and a meat-centered diet—and the wages to pay for it—as their American right.[41]

The right to meat and the fight for adequate wages, therefore, became intertwined. The profession of nutrition emerged to negotiate this struggle, between industrialists seeking to keep wages in check by urging workers to eat less and cheaper cuts of meat and workers who saw a meat-centered diet as part of the American promise. Using the recently discovered science of calories and animal feeding experiments, an emerging group of nutrition professionals demonstrated that the American diet contained just about too much of everything at too much cost. University professor W. O. Atwater became the authority on how much food was necessary for workers. He established the first food laboratories and eventually led the first Department of Agricultural Experiment Stations at the US Department of Agriculture (USDA). Even before his USDA appointment, Atwater had been using his scientific research to formulate a set of eating standards he published for popular consumption in various magazines. In his role as a USDA official, this advice became the first official US dietary standards, in 1894.[42] While much of his popular dietary advice had to do with curing the ills of magazine readers, generally the dyspeptic middle class, he also turned his attention to wageworkers and how much they needed to be fed to perform work.

In these articles, Atwater described his work on "a pecuniary economy of food"; specifically, "How much protein, fats, and carbohydrates does the average man, with a moderate amount of manual work to do, require in a day's food?" For the antebellum Grahamites of the early nineteenth century, "luxury" foods defined ill-health and bad morals. For Gilded Age industrial-ists and nutritionists, meat-eating represented something else: the "waste" of higher wages. At the center of Atwater's advice, therefore, was the idea of eating some meat but not too much, and of determining what now is known as "the best value for the dollar" in terms of buying cheap cuts of meat. He castigated workers who bought higher quality than they could afford. In his argument in favor of a more pecuniary workers' economy, he featured the story of a coal miner who "was innocently committing an immense economi-cal and hygienic blunder" through his "conceit . . . that there is some mysteri-ous virtue in those kinds of food that have the most delicate appearance and flavor and the highest price . . . and that to economize by using anything inferior would be a sacrifice of both dignity and principle."[43] The emphasis in Atwater's nutritional studies was on adequate and efficient intake to fuel the worker's bodily machine.

Surprisingly, the bridge between industry and reform is once again Edward Atkinson, John Brown supporter and free market ideologue who had opposed slavery because it was inefficient and who had helped create the sharecropping system. He opposed meat-heavy diets for workers as inefficient fuel for the human machine. Atkinson, like his antebellum colleagues, was (at least by the time of his obituary) a vegetarian, but his reasons for rejecting meat, like his reasons for rejecting slavery and for rejecting redistribution of land to freed slaves, was efficiency. To do this, Atkinson became a major supporter of Atwater and of the founder of home economics, Ellen Swallow Richards. Richards, the first female MIT professor, sought to establish home economics as a profession that would inculcate efficiency into American eating and other household activities. Atkinson helped Richards's and her partner, Mary Hinman Abel, to establish the New England Kitchen. Abel described this establishment as "an experiment to determine the successful conditions of preparing, by scientific methods, from the cheaper food materials, nutritious and palatable dishes, which should find a ready demand at paying prices."[44] The New England Kitchen meals were designed to provide adequate calories most efficiently: in this pre-vitamin era, that meant cheaper cuts of meat, without vegetables, with sweetened condensed milk and white flour as cheap sources of carbohydrates and protein.[45]

Supported by Atkinson, nutritionists transformed the fight between workers and industrialists over a "living wage" to a question of how much a worker needed to live, a conversation between workers and these professionals rather than workers and their employers. To further his project of dietary efficiency, Atkinson had invented a new oven—the Aladdin Oven—that cooked food using only a kerosene lamp. The oven may have been efficient from a fuel perspective, but it was dangerous and took hours to heat and to cook the food.[46]

In other words, one of the first tasks taken on by nutrition as an emerging profession was to delegitimize workers' demands for more. Atwater's scientific claims against workers relied on a new scientific measure: the calorie. Atwater trained in Europe, where German scientists first discovered a way to measure the calories provided by food and, in turn, the calories needed by people to perform various kinds of work. Bringing this knowledge back to the United States, Atwater found that American workers ate both more protein and more calories than the workers of Germany at the time. Atwater assumed this was due to greater activity in US workers—that they worked harder—but also to a mistaken love of rich foods on the part of the country's working classes.[47]

Workers in Europe may have been malnourished but American workers, according to Atwater, ate too much. Atwater's pecuniary economy saw the worker's body as an efficient machine—"The steam-engine gets its power from fuel; the body does the same"—and his mission was to determine how to "fuel the body" as cheaply as possible.[48] In this way, the Yankee notion of productive labor became open to the scientific measurement of efficiency.

But behind this machine metaphor was a struggle between bettering society by making it more efficient versus the workers' claim that a better society could be achieved through economic redistribution by way of higher wages. As the working class demanded higher wages, nutritionists and other new professionals, deploying science, designed counterarguments to show how efficiency in the home could maintain social reproduction at lower income. The nutrition professionals argued that workers did not need higher wages but rather more discipline in their food budgets.[49]

Leaders of the workers' unions saw the dietary studies as an aggressive counterattack against their demand for higher wages. Working-class leaders like Eugene Debs and Samuel Gompers opposed Atkinson's ideas about food, referring to him as "Shinbone Atkinson" because he advocated cheaper cuts of meat for workers, which seemed to come down to the boiling of bones. Yet, the union leaders' response to the attack on workers' demands for a meat-eating wage was not against nutritionists but against an ethnic group that ate less meat: the Chinese.

RACIAL GUT WARS

In 1901 Samuel Gompers and American Federation of Labor leader Herman Gudstadt published a pamphlet: "Some Reasons for Chinese Exclusion: Meat vs. Rice: American Manhood vs. Asiatic Coolieism—Which Will Survive?" Gompers and Gudstadt wrote the pamphlet in support of extending the 1882 Chinese Exclusion Act, which severely restricted Chinese immigration into the country. Surprisingly, they made known their sentiments about Chinese immigration in terms of the Chinese rice-centered diet: "He underbids all white labor and ruthlessly takes its place and will go on doing so until the white laborer comes down to the scanty food and half-civilized habits of the Chinaman." Much of the report is filled with fears of crime and disease, an appeal to middle-class fears of contagion. But these labor organizers also saw Chinese immigrants' cheaper, rice-centered diets—and their supposed willingness to accept lower wages because of this cheaper diet—as a threat to their right to meat.[50]

Yet, the American popular media was both fascinated and repelled by Chinese habits. For example in 1889, *Current Literature,* a kind of pre–*Reader's Digest*, printed a piece about everyday Chinese life. The article praises Chinese dietary habits: "The universal diet consists of rice, beans, millet, garden vegetables, and fish, with a little meat on high festivals. Wholesome food in abundance may be supplied at less than a penny a day for each adult, and even in famine times thousands of persons have been kept alive for months on about half a penny a day each." The article ends with a story of an old Chinese woman who was so concerned about wasting others' labor that she tried to walk her way to the cemetery before she died.[51]

For those Americans who maintained the moral rectitude of discipline and self-denial, the Chinese lifestyle was a remarkable reminder of what discipline looked like. For industrialists, such as Central Pacific Railroad member and construction contractor Charles Crocker, the Chinese were admirable for their "steadiness, and the aptitude and capacity for hard work."[52] The Central Pacific rail line construction at the time employed as many as ten thousand Chinese workers. In San Francisco shoe factories, employers paid Chinese laborers a third of white wages. For the industrialists, the Chinese were an admirably efficient working force.[53]

White workers, who saw themselves in competition with Chinese workers, did not agree: "They routinely attempted to create, extend, or preserve their social position against the perceived threat that the Chinese posed to their superordinate status."[54] Diet became one of the arenas of struggle over racial superiority. Rejecting both industrialist and middle-class interest in the Chinese as the disciplined worker, as well as nutritionists' arguments that their meat-centered diet was overly luxurious, worker representatives struck back, on behalf of both meat and native working-class interests. Worker organizer Eugene Debs also used the Chinese diet in his opposition to Atwater, Atkinson, and Richards's investigations into worker nutrition efficiencies. In an 1892 letter to Atkinson, Debs asks for "your lowest estimate of the cost of a 'square meal' for a working-man." Ironically admitting that "you have succeeded in demonstrating that an American laborer, by scientific methods, can feed himself at a cost as low as Chinamen are subjected to," Debs asked Atkinson to give him a list of foods in this diet.[55]

Yet, the truly threatening aspect of the Chinese presence in America was not about disease or diet but about discipline. In fact, Gompers's description of the Chinese "character" ironically sounds much like the type of person the Yankee reformers were trying to bring forth: "endowed with untiring industry; temperate to the utmost abstemiousness; frugal; a born merchant; a first class cultivator, especially in gardening; distinguished in every kind of handicraft, the son of the Middle Kingdom slowly, surely and unremarked is supplanting the Europeans wherever they are brought together."[56] Therefore, even within this anti-immigration tract, the representation of Chinese racial subjectivity vacillates between degradation and discipline. One side of the story painted the presence of the Chinese as entirely of disease and want, of a people who had learned to make do with less because they had to, who were now competing with those who had had the benefit of more. As a result, the Chinese lifestyle, but especially diet, was considered unnatural, unmanly, and un-American. In the West, municipal authorities used sanitary regulations to try to eliminate Chinese vegetable merchants in the cities, a business that clearly grew out of the needs of the more vegetable-intensive Chinese diet.[57] From the American Federation of Labor perspective, what nutritionists like Atwater were trying to do was to make the American worker more like the Asian one. The Chinese worker became tangled up in national wage struggles, serving as a double icon of both discipline and degradation. The message mixed real issues of poverty—places where people were so poor they supposedly only eat rice—with ideas of national worker deservedness.

From the Gilded Age workers' perspective, the "What to eat?" question was about the right to be an American citizen deserving of comfort, not the antebellum virtuous citizen eating abstemiously to bring God's perfection to earth. To the working class, the Chinese and their diet became the representation of the type of abstemious life reformers wanted workers to live, if they accepted both the idea of self-discipline and the physical presence of Chinese immigrants that would force them to eat this way. Gompers argued that the Chinese diet created a situation in which "their ability to subsist and thrive under conditions that would mean starvation and suicide to the cheapest worker of Europe" points to an already-set social agreement about an American standard of living that was more than just enough.[58]

The question "What to eat?" therefore became increasingly tied up with cultural ideas of morality that affected struggles among workers. The workers' narrative of American exceptionalism was of pride to live in a country where they got more than enough, where a living wage brought more than sufficiency, allowing workers a modicum of comfort. "What the average American ate never failed to fascinate foreign sojourners," Arthur Schlesinger states in his article "A Dietary Interpretation of American History": "Coming from lands where the growth of population constantly pressed upon the means of subsistence, they marveled at the profusion and variety of dishes which the American regarded as his birthright."[59] At the center of that birthright was meat.

Unfortunately, this American exceptionalism entailed a stigmatization of other diets, including one that contained some very worthwhile elements: grains, vegetables, and, in particular, fiber. The Union triumph in the Civil War made the Northern European diet, centered around meat and milk, the American Ideal. While nutritionists advised cheap cuts of meat, there was no questioning the basic components of the meal—meat, milk, and flour. Vegetables, particularly greens, as well as beans and rice, were dietary elements associated with stigmatized groups. Meat and potatoes became the paragon of the American exceptionalist ideal, a diet that workers deserved and defended.

FREE TO EAT

For the industrial elite, however, the Gilded Age was a time for overindulgence rather than discipline. Consumer culture became the culture of comfort, with the tempting claim that "material and moral developments were but two sides of the same coin."[60] Consumption became, as Thorstein Veblen observed, the "conspicuous" signifier of deservedness. Harvey Levenstein's history of US eating habits tells very well the story of what the Gilded Age upper classes actually ate: for the most part, too much. The elite preached a sermon of moderation to workers while themselves embracing the "spirit of gluttony" that so frustrated Graham earlier in the century. The "fat cat" was a sign of the successful consumer, the one who could live a life of luxury and comfort, a consumer dream of indulgence without consequences. Millionaires competed to be the most lavish in their entertainments, the winner probably being the elaborate dinner put on by wealthy gas magnate and horse enthusiast C. K. G. Billings, who invited guests to dine while seated on horses, with waiters dressed like grooms. In ingestive displays such as this $50,000 affair, girth rather than self-control became the sign of success. The Southern notions of food as comfort became the elite ideal of conspicuous consumption.

Workers struggled against industrialist attempts to change their diets, and at the same time joined their employers in the desire for comfort and consumption as signs of success. To be able to consume freely became the sign of personal autonomy, a consumer citizenship not influenced by or dependent on others: "I'd rather eat what I'd rather. I don't want to eat what's good for me," one woman purportedly said in response to the rather bland food served at the New England Kitchen.[61]

Workers turned away from efficient consumption and toward the achievement of comfort as the American ideal: greater girth, more leisure time, higher wages, more consumer goods, and, in particular, meat. The notion of dietary citizenship rejected the nutritionist professionals' call for a more "pecuniary" lifestyle and instead embraced an American exceptionalist consumer rhetoric representing the nation's citizens as deserving of more than mere survival.

Immigrants also rejected the cultural domination of the Kitchen's predominantly New England dishes such as "Pilgrim succotash" and creamed codfish. Boston's immigrant poor rejected the food Richards and Abel offered, seeing it as a form of cultural domination. Refusing to eat the Indian pudding on the New England Kitchen menu, one man commented: "You needn't try to make a Yankee of me by making me eat that."[62]

Workers also rejected nutritionists' claims that their carefully designed recipes were healthier. A commercial product—the laxative—emerged to help resolve the tension between health and comfort, between "eating what I want" and the "eating what you should" claims of nutritionists. Overeaters made up for their indulgence in all sorts of disturbing ways: mercury pills, intestinal operations, strange diets, and constant enemas, like the nineteenth-century woman who testified that, when running from her burning home, she made sure to take one thing: her Cascade enema bag.[63] The Gilded Age dyspepsia advertisements in Figure 3 show how companies claimed to overcome the tension between eating and health. Laxative, diet, and dyspepsia advertising claimed to give the overindulgent consumer the ability to break dietary rules with impunity: "no dieting," "no purge," "no starving," and the almost constant phrase: "eat what you please." These ads, typical of dyspepsia, obesity, and laxative ads of the time, often featured testimonials by individuals stating that the product enabled them to "eat what I want."

In these stories, the purchase of a commercial product promised to give the consumer the physical effects of discipline without the need for self-control. Yet, despite their promises, laxative products did not resolve these tensions. Stomach ailments were such a common torment at the time that even health reformer and cereal tycoon C. W. Post was eventually driven to give up on Grape-Nuts as a cure for his stomach pains and took his own life with a shotgun.[64] Bad middle-class stomachs and bad working-class wages formed an ironic tangle of interests that underlay "What to eat?" rhetoric. Yet, despite the material realities—low wages and indigestion—answers to the "What to eat?" question reflected a kind of cultural supremacy, justifying the ways of life of some over others. Progressive food reformers emerged to negotiate these class, race, and ethnic tensions, although not always successfully. As the next chapter will show, out of these tensions emerged a Progressive professional class that solidified a new narrative about good eating and social order.

4

Pure Food and the Progressive Body

NO ONE READS HERBERT SPENCER any more. Yet, he was *the* social philosopher of the late nineteenth century, widely read, formulating an idea of society that pervaded public thought and action of the time. He had an enormous influence on the sociologist Emile Durkheim, and through Durkheim and others, continues to influence ideas about social life. An autodidact who lived off the income from his writings, Spencer read everything, from biology to history to anthropology. From his reading, Spencer sought to formulate a unified theory of social change. To do this, he studied the organization of simple organisms and the changes that occurred as organisms became more complex. He began writing about these ideas just before Darwin, and then later translated Darwin's biological ideas of natural selection into a concept of social change he called "the survival of the fittest."

Spencer viewed society as a body and used evolutionary concepts of increasing biological complexity to describe social change. The overarching idea by which Spencer sought to unify all theories of existence was the organism—the body. Spencer studied organisms from the most simple to the most complex and posited a theory of society based on the ways in which organisms became more complex by differentiating their functions. In his article "The Social Organism," Spencer describes how, as organisms become more complex, cells differentiate between alimentary and regulatory functions. For Spencer, the same process happens in society, as "the elaboration and distribution of nutriment, or of commodities, is a necessary accompaniment of further differentiation of functions in the individual body or in the body-politic."[1] While other philosophers, such as Plato and Hobbes, had used the body as a metaphor for society, Spencer used evolutionary biology to formulate an overall theory that explained all forms of social life.

Commodities became the blood and food the viscera that supported the higher forms of the system. Those who provided food for the social system—workers—remained primitive, like the primitive cells of simple organisms that become part of digestive systems in more complex organisms. These digestive cells functioned to support higher, more complex forms of life, the upper classes. Spencer's ideas of the body-politic became the major metaphor to explain the emergence of social classes in industrial society. Durkheim took these ideas and elaborated them into a more communal idea of society as a body composed of differentiated but mutually supportive organs, all of which were dependent on the other organs for their existence. These ideas made the body one of the major metaphors of the twentieth century.

An emerging group of American professionals took up these European ideas and incorporated them into American ideas of society as a self-controlled body. Scientists, experts, government officials, and industrialists saw themselves as taking on the role of managing society. Individuals performed roles that contributed to the social whole the way organs function in the body. For Progressives, the health of this social body, composed of groups such as unions, government, business, agriculture, and professional associations, depended on scientific expertise. Like the virtuous civic republican body, the virtuous social body required control. Progressive experts saw themselves as the creators of these new forms of social control, creating a better society: "through adherence to scientific principles ... to identify the most desirable ends to be achieved."[2] They did this as the growing industrial economy brought into the country more workers from Eastern and Southern Europe, whose cultures and practices spelled danger to those wanting to maintain an American national character.

Experts used the language of science and economics to advocate for new organizational controls. Trust in science and rational planning became the mediating solution to political conflicts: farmers would prosper with scientifically improved agriculture, businesses would become more efficient and profitable and stable, and the workforce would learn its role.[3] For example, agricultural experts argued that efficient organization would solve farmers' inability to control the prices they received for their crops and livestock. Industry experts argued that businesses could be efficiently organized to control workers on the factory floor. And experts working for unions argued that efficient and centralized union organization was the best way to exact better working conditions from employers. Finally, the new class of nutrition experts argued that a well-organized diet would lead to a healthier American population.

Progressive ideas about society as a body broke down the working-class resistance to control by experts. Historian Robert Wiebe has argued that the twentieth century brought "a new structure of loyalties to replace the decaying system of the nineteenth-century communities."[4] Scientific experts became the voice of the mainstream narrative about freedom and order in American society.[5] This new scientific class "found their rewards more and more in the uniqueness of an occupation and in its importance to a rising scientific-industrial society."[6] Increasingly, Progressive Era reformers saw the expert—often in government or academia—as the manager, the brain, of this larger social body: "his vision encompassed the entire nation, his impartiality freed him from all prejudices, and his detached wisdom enabled him to devise an equitable and progressive policy for the whole society."[7]

The focus of much of the scientific language used by this new class of professionals was purity. Like earlier reformers, they categorized what was pure and what was not, yet in this case through the authority of scientific expertise, developed through new organizational capacities like government agencies and universities. In the building of the federal state populated by scientific expertise, the search for purity focused particularly on food.

Central to the Progressive Era's dietary reforms was the discovery of the germ. The acceptance of germ theory late in the nineteenth century[8] brought new public fears of contamination as well as a deeper awareness of the real urban diseases that threatened, in particular, children. Like the angels that revealed new diets during the Second Great Awakening,[9] germs were not visible to the naked eye, and thus needed the intervention of humans with a special gift of vision. Scientists and public health professionals became the new visionaries. Germs, therefore, like angels, enabled a particular class to claim authority and to embrace purity as something that excluded those who did not adopt a particular way of life. Through the vision of scientific sanitary and nutritional expertise, middle-class fear of dirt, germs, and contamination led to new forms of purification—suburbs, eugenics, disinfectants.[10]

By the 1890s, the germ theory of disease had taken hold. Housewives had, since the mid-1800s, been warned to maintain cleanliness against the threat of "ferments" or "miasmas" which caused disease, but only at the end of the century was it widely accepted that these threats were not chemical but biological. Miasmas were understood to be visible as dust and perceivable as smells; microbes, however, were not detectable without special instruments and skills, leaving women dependent on scientific advice to maintain this more intense form of household purification. Nancy Tomes argues that this transformation of household sanitation paralleled similar changes in municipal public health institutions. Housewives became sanitarians and housekeeping became a scientific vocation that welcomed female expertise: "Sweeping and cleaning and laundry work are all processes of sanitation and not mere drudgery," explained one of these first female experts, Ellen Swallow Richards.[11] Through academic classes and as agricultural extension agents, these new home economics professionals taught the science of housekeeping to women anxious to avoid illness in their families. One of the major ways that middle- and upper-class women perceived their responsibilities in keeping their family safe from disease was to put stronger boundaries between their families and those outside.

Along with new public sanitation measures and the development of antibiotics, these changed practices had real effects that lowered death rates from contagious diseases. By developing sanitary infrastructure and policies in cities, the new professionals affected mortality, particularly infant mortality. Yet, the metaphor of the body threatened by contagion went beyond protecting the household to the larger project of protecting the nation from foreign genes, germs, and foods: "contagion and (national) culture were mutually constituted terms even before late-nineteenth-century bacteriology made the microbe a popular topic of national inquiry and debate," yet the cultural change caused by the emergence of bacteriology as a science "was dramatic."[12] Food purity became wrapped up with ideas of purifying society through social control of environment and behavior. Sanitarians (mis-)interpreted the new science of human ecology—understanding the link between humans and their environment—as a motivation to "secure boundaries: boundaries of the home, the body, and the nation, as infectious agents threatened to obliterate these borders."[13] Ideas about good food followed suit: advertisements and government bulletins increasingly described good food as pure food, free of "adulteration." Government scientist Harvey Wiley muckraked in the popular press against adulterated food and drink, but it took the description of factory contamination in Upton Sinclair's *The Jungle* to generate public support for the legislation that became the Pure Food and Drug Act of 1906.

Another aspect of American lives that had become invisible was the structure of the new industrial, modern economy itself. Americans, "whose powers of economic decision had been expropriated by the system of corporate organization," became increasingly unsettled about an economy based on the investment of their savings rather than their own personal proprietorship.[14] As consumers, they became increasingly dependent on regulations and expertise to indicate which foods and medicines were truly healthy and which were "adulterated." The discovery of vitamins brought a new class of experts who measured the nutritional benefits of particular foods and provided advice on the "right" diet based on those measurements.

Germs, vitamins, and modern economics—all invisible to the naked eye—encouraged the view of a healthy society as one, interdependent body dependent on experts to "see" good health. As a result, "reluctantly rather than enthusiastically, the average American tended more and more to rely on government regulation, to seek in governmental action a counterpoise to the power of private business."[15] Academic intellectuals took up this banner, arguing that science and expertise would "ensure the development of a moral society, in which the social instinct is cultivated and self-interest made to comport with freedom of action," ideas about moral citizenship that would have been familiar to Benjamin Rush. To do this, experts argued, "it may be necessary for the State to interfere with individual freedom of action, to condition the individual, through education and, if necessary, coercion, to behave in the common interest."[16] As a result, education reform, legislation, and dietary reform mixed together with other Progressive plans for creating this new healthy mass citizenry.

One of the ideals Progressive reformers sought was the perfect body. Harvard anthropometry expert Dudley Allen Sargent measured thousands of bodies to discover the golden mean of physical health and beauty. Sargent, whose "tests emerged as one of the most common schemes for judging group and individual development," determined the ideal strength and size of the human body at the fiftieth percentile of his measurements, which he described as "perfect symmetry."[17] Unable to find such ideal bodies in real life, Sargent had sculptures made to represent this golden mean for the 1893 World Exposition in Chicago, to "show what might be called typically healthy Americans, or the symmetry of perfect normalcy."[18]

In the same way, politically "the Progressives stood for a dual program of economic remedies designed to minimize the dangers from the extreme left and right."[19] Theodore Roosevelt represented the golden mean in government, wary of both "the purblind folly of the very rich men; their greed and arrogance" as well as "a very unhealthy condition of excitement and irritation in the popular mind, which shows itself in part in the enormous increase in the socialistic propaganda," such as Sinclair's *The Jungle* and the muckraking magazines.[20] Much like Graham's ideas of healthy food in previous decades, Roosevelt and the new middle-class governmental and academic experts saw themselves as representing the moderate political mean between too much and too little political stimulation. But the golden mean, much like older temperance ideas, overlapped in the minds of Progressive health reformers with ideas of perfect cleanliness. Purity became the norm and cleanliness the sign of health. Health reformers therefore became what James Whorton calls "hygiene ideologues" advocating a pure way of life that centered on ideas of both sanitation and efficiency.[21]

HYGIENE IDEOLOGUES

The rise of the mass-market magazine, made affordable by new printing technologies, the lowering of postal rates, and the development of advertising created a new mass reading public. The Northeastern print culture, much of which emerged from the Yankee reformer's need for a didactic platform, became the national voice of this new mass public. In these publications, muckraking journalists both created a more informed public and produced a new set of broad anxieties about healthy living.[22] Despite Progressive reformers' ideas that they were the moderating force in a society torn by extremes, the actual line between muckraker and professional expert at this time was unclear. Many of those writing about the adulteration of food and drugs were civic or government officials working to pass legislation to regulate food products and patent medicines. Others were reformers belonging to groups agitating for regulation that would put food production in the control of experts. And both of these groups spoke loudly to the press about the importance of purity.

Ellen Swallow Richards, Harvey Wiley, Irving Fisher, John Harvey Kellogg, Horace Fletcher, and Elie Metchnikoff were some of the most popular writer-experts addressing a mass public about eating and health. These experts were social reformers in government, academia, and private industry. Unlike the vegetarians and nutritionists of the nineteenth century, these reformers were prominent members of established American institutions. They used their place in those institutions to change popular opinion about good living.

The work of many of these reformers spanned the Gilded Age into the Progressive Era. Ellen Swallow Richards's 1880s book, *The Chemistry of*

Cooking and Cleaning: A Manual for Housekeepers, is more in the style of the Beechers, while her 1904 work, *The Art of Right Living,* exemplifies the expansion of the role of the expert in managing everyday life habits. Also, despite their different disciplines, most of the Progressive expert-reformers came from Yankee backgrounds. Most were raised in middle-class Northeastern religious families with a high moral culture. As a result, most mixed professional concerns with moral concerns and saw their work as a moral mission. Like the earlier reformers, they believed in the print culture of didactic exhortation and wrote popular works for this new mass public on how to live well. This moral mission encouraged Progressive reformers to combine proven scientific discoveries with a set of pseudoscientific mis-discoveries about society. Food reformers in particular used unproven ideas about nutrition to create an idea of perfect eating.

Home economics as a profession emerged from this Progressive reform movement. Cooking advice moved from the Boston and New York Cooking Schools to academic departments, housed primarily in Northeastern institutions. Richards, the first woman in America to receive a chemistry degree, as well as the first woman professor at MIT, initiated yearly meetings for home economics professionals beginning in 1898, in Lake Placid, New York. Established at the Lake Placid Conferences, home economics put professional women like Richards in charge of improving the population through behavioral change. Home economics set curricula for teaching what Richards called "euthenics": "[t]he betterment of living conditions, through conscious endeavor, for the purpose of securing efficient human beings."[23] Richards meant to provide an alternative to eugenics through the purification of a population's environment and behavior rather than through the eugenetic practice of sterilizing the "unfit." Yet, Richards's definition of right living was still based on the establishment of an ideal, in this case an ideal environment and way of life rather than the ideal of genetic fitness.

Richards's leadership, based on New England culture, especially its diet, solidified Yankee Northern European culture as the definition of what good American living should be, including good American eating. Richards's earlier 1890s project, the New England Kitchen, was part of her project of euthenics. Yet, the New England Kitchen "failed to change the eating habits of Boston's poor."[24] Learning from this failure, Richards decided the solution was to establish home economics as a profession, spreading from her narrower "chemistry of cleaning" and efficient eating base to broad social "right living" reform. As home economics transitioned from cooking, clean-

ing, and childcare advice to the larger stage of "municipal housekeeping"—
what temperance reformer Frances Willard called "housekeeping on the
broadest scale"—the New England ideal of Yankee culture once again provided the model of a good and healthy life.[25]

Rather than discovering good foods, Harvey Wiley's mission was
to uncover the adulteration of food by invisible chemical compounds that
industrial food processors used to either preserve or extend foods. Wiley
was originally skeptical about using the press to forward his goals. However,
the public became fascinated with Wiley's experiments with the Poison
Squad, a group of volunteer civil service employees who tested the effects of
various preservatives by eating them in daily meals. This convinced him to use
newspaper coverage of these experiments as a way to promote concern about
food adulteration. Along with Upton Sinclair's *The Jungle* this publicity
helped pass the Pure Food and Drug Act of 1906. Wiley later moved from his
government position to head the health section of *Good Housekeeping,* becoming one of the prime popular didactic voices on food and health in the mass
media.[26]

The academic Irving Fisher was another widely read expert whose mission
was dietary reform. At the turn of the twentieth century, Fisher was the
nation's most-cited economist.[27] Like many Progressive reformers, he was a
child of strict religious upbringing who combined ideas of efficiency and a
gospel of self-control. He promoted vegetarian eating in his popular book,
How to Live (1915), a best-seller at 400,000 copies in twenty-one editions, and
was one of the first to propound calorie counting as the foundation of healthy
eating. His work on calories paralleled his disciplinary work on the economics of utility. One of the first to employ mathematics to measure economic
efficiency, Fisher's measurement of calories in food reflected his interest in
the measurement of utility in economics.[28]

Horace Fletcher, neither academic nor public official, was a popular writer
for the mass public, formulating a new cult of optimism that found inspiration in new ideas about living efficiently as a way to perfect humanity. Fletcher
is known for his advocacy of mastication—100 chews before swallowing—but
this was just part of an overall regimen of efficient eating that lowered the
amount of protein and total food ingested. For Fletcher, the telltale indication
of efficient eating was negligible bowel movements that "had no more odor
than a hot biscuit."[29] For Fletcher, chewing was the link between efficiency
and health, since fully chewed food enabled the body to efficiently digest the
complete nutrition in food. These claims gained the attention of economists

at Yale University, including Irving Fisher, who brought Fletcher to New Haven and performed exercise experiments on him and others who ate his highly chewed low-protein meals.

John Harvey Kellogg's Battle Creek sanatorium mostly served the wealthy who suffered from the effects of their food indulgences. With the help of his brother, Will Keith, Kellogg developed the sanatorium from a religious mission into a mass-market food company. Kellogg also propounded his ideas to a larger mass audience in books and his own magazine, *Good Health*. He became the sanatorium director through his membership in the Seventh-day Adventists and was personally appointed by the founders Helen G. and James White. Although the sanatorium later separated from this religious community, Kellogg's dietary recommendations closely followed the Seventh-day Adventist beliefs about vegetarianism and personal purity. Kellogg's own ideas about lowering meat in the diet agreed with Fletcher's, and he added the ideas about mastication to his eating advice at Battle Creek. Unlike Fletcher, however, who had lived in Asia, admired the Japanese, and may have taken some of his ideas about low-protein eating from the Asian diet, Kellogg linked ideas about dietary efficiency with ideas of racial purity. With Fisher, Kellogg founded the main eugenic society of the day, the Race Betterment Foundation, of which Wiley was a member. Even Richards, while emphasizing euthenics, gave credence to eugenic notions as well.[30]

Hygienic ideology linked to the idea of society as a body and purity as a mission meant that a health panic about germs and genes was linked to a moral panic about social virtues and a hope that government could better both health and morals through policies that sanitized and purified American society. Progressive dietary advice became a narrative of how to protect the individual's threatened body from itself (see figure 5). Modern medicine rose to protect that body, beginning with the concept of miasmas, then advancing to germ theory and ultimately to the discovery of immunity by Elie Metchnikoff. Metchnikoff was the first to recognize that certain cells in the body—the phagocytes—worked specifically to rid the body of infectious bacteria by eating them. The idea of the body as defended by internal immunity required a new narrative about the body and its relationship to the world.[31] Metchnikoff won the Nobel Prize for his discovery. His work on the macrophages' role in immunity envisioned the body as under attack by outside sources, and withstanding these attacks through its own internal defense system. In this narrative, immunity thereby becomes a bodily garrison ready for war. A highly bounded and militarized body became the modern medical

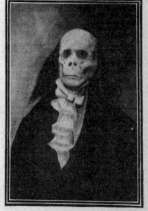

INDIANA
STATE BOARD *of* HEALTH

I AM
DEATH

**TO EARLY JOIN ME
BREATHE MUCH
FOUL AIR,
DRINK ALCOHOLIC
LIQUORS,
EAT MIDNIGHT SUPPERS,
EAT LOTS OF RICH FOOD,
BOLT YOUR FOOD OR WASH IT DOWN
WITH LARGE AMOUNTS OF
BLACK COFFEE,
NEGLECT YOUR BOWELS.**

FIGURE 5. Indiana State Board of Health advertisement. Indiana State Board of Health. *Monthly Bulletin* 15, no. 4 (1912): 40. Courtesy Ruth Lilly Memorial Library, Indiana University.

view of health. Metchnikoff's ideas finalized the boundary-building between the body and the world.

But Metchnikoff had greater ambitions than the simple healing of wounds: his mission was to prolong life itself. In that quest, as he explains in his 1908 book *The Prolongation of Life,* he turned to the colon, which he saw as a vestige of an earlier evolutionary adaptation, with us but no longer necessary. This organ, he theorized, becomes clogged with undigested food that sits and ferments, poisoning the body with its fermented chemicals, a process he called "autointoxication." An idea that first emerged in ancient Egypt, it was widely shared by the medical experts in Metchnikoff's time. The ancient rationale around autointoxication was that the intestinal boundary between fecal matter and blood was suspect. Fecal dirt needed to be flushed out before its toxic matter leaked through the walls and into the blood system.[32] Some argued that the solution was a kind of mega-enema that cleans the toxins from the colon. Others recommended a surgical solution: the removal of the colon itself, a particularly dangerous solution in the pre-germ theory surgical era. Metchnikoff had a more gentle solution: to ingest a beneficial microbe to colonize the colon, a strain of *Lactobacillus Bulgaricus* that came from certain fermented milks drunk by supposedly long-lived Bulgarians, which would neutralize the internal toxicity.

Metchnikoff's story about *L. Bulgaricus* was a narrative of bodily repair in which humans ally with certain organisms to fight bad intruders: he spoke of beneficial bacteria as soldiers on the intestinal battlefield, doing work at the bacterial level much like phagocytes did for cells.[33] In Metchnikoff's martial story, lactic acid bacteria—supposedly the "good" colon bacteria—produce peroxide to kill off other kinds of "germs." The result is a kind of bacterial purification that eliminates corruption from the body. Therefore, a healthy colon is one occupied by bacteria friendly to the body but dangerous to its enemies, a kind of internal garrison in which the colonization becomes the metaphor to describe the healthy colon.

Elie Metchnikoff and his ideas about digestion arrived at the Pasteur Institute in Paris early in the twentieth century and then into the diets of food reformers such as John Harvey Kellogg. Ambitious entrepreneurs made pilgrimages to the Pasteur Institute to fetch *L. Bulgaricus* and return to their countries to make yogurt. These aspiring businessmen included Isaac Carasso, who, according to a company history, traveled from Spain to obtain Metchnikoff's purified strains of *L. Bulgaricus* for the new yogurt company he named after his son: Danone.[34]

DIETARY EUGENICS

The public depended on experts to explain the role of another invisible agent: the gene. In the early decades of the twentieth century, the link between social reform as the improvement of the social body, and the genetics behind the creation of individual bodies, led many Progressives to eugenic ideas.

The founders of American sociology, Charles Cooley, Lester Ward, and Edward Ross, all believed in controlling reproduction, environment, and behavior for the purpose of "race betterment." First coined by Francis Galton in 1883 as "the science of improving stock," [35] this project of social purification encompassed both direct issues of who reproduced with whom—the "hard" genetics of sterilization—and the "softer genetics" of governmental policies that "give the more suitable races or strains of blood a better chance." [36] Minimum wage policy, for example, was born as a form of eugenics policy— the belief that only the fittest would be hired at these higher wages and degenerate laborers would lose their access to livelihood and therefore fail to reproduce. Socialist economists such as Richard Ely, while focusing primarily on government control of the environment, believed that "degeneracy" could be eliminated from the human population through control of reproduction. Many eugenicists saw the problem as providing charity to the poor for their survival, enabling the "less fit" to reproduce. Others were more concerned about immigration, focusing on the flow of recent immigrants from Southern and Eastern Europe, who were seen as diluting the "native stock" by their greater fertility, leading to "race suicide." [37]

Many Progressive advocated the more extreme solution: the forced sterilization of "defectives." Progressives advocated for government control to separate out those who deserved to reproduce from those who were, through soft discouragement or hard means like sterilization, kept from reproducing the next generation. Justice Oliver Wendell Holmes, in his Supreme Court opinion advocating forced sterilization, justified it as a benefit to society at large: "It is better for all the world, if instead of waiting to execute degenerate offspring for crime or to let them starve for their imbecility, society can prevent those who are manifestly unfit from continuing their kind.... Three generations of imbeciles are enough." [38]

While "the term eugenics encompassed a large and shifting constellation of meanings," the movement "mixed specifically genetic concerns with a much broader range of preventive health measures, including personal and public hygiene, diet, and exercise." [39] Progressives seeking to change personal behaviors and environment, like Richards and Wiley, saw these softer "euthenic" policies as short-term prescriptions to foster positive change while waiting for the longer-term policies of eugenics to take hold. Richards defined eugenics as "hygiene for future generations," while euthenics was "hygiene for the present generation." [40] While one involved education, government regulation, and public health initiatives, and the other involved forced sterilization and the separation of the population into pure and degenerate, both relied on a notion of purity as the creation of an ideal and the setting of strong boundaries between those who fit the ideal and those who needed to be either eliminated from, or educated toward, that ideal.

Therefore, many Progressives saw morality, eugenics, and food purity as going hand in hand. Harvey Washington Wiley, the central figure in the passage of the Pure Food and Drug Act of 1906, and subsequently head of the new Food and Drug Administration, mixed pure food advocacy with moral exhortations and eugenic beliefs. In his congressional testimony in favor of the Pure Food and Drug Act, he called food fraud "demoralizing" to business: "No man can continually deceive his customer and retain that high moral sense which is the very soul of trade."[41] He was also active in the Conferences for Race Betterment, founded by John Harvey Kellogg, who funded the Race Betterment Foundation from his corn-flake profits. Others, such as Medical Association of Georgia President W. B. Hardman, addressing the association's 1914 annual meeting, praised the passage of the Pure Food and Drug Act as part of the "social gospel," but stated that the most important aspect of that gospel was "eugenic laws, so that the creature of the future may be a better specimen of manhood and womanhood."[42] Margaret Sanger, Upton Sinclair, H. G. Wells, and other prominent Progressives sanctioned eugenic policies.

But, in the end, purity meant "absence": "an absence from meat of the nauseating ingredients Sinclair had alleged, an absence from processed food of the poisonous preservatives Wiley had condemned, an absence from patent medicines of the dangerous narcotics," all contaminants that prompted "shock and fear."[43] And while public health Progressives got involved in state-level eugenic sterilization policies that affected thousands of people, their real impact in promoting social "absence" was through anti-immigration policies and the Jim Crow policies of the post-Reconstruction South. Studies showing that immigrants and blacks were of shorter stature and more prone to contagious diseases were also arguments for absence.

MILK, MEAT, AND RACE

World War I brought to the fore the need for strong soldiers' bodies. Nutrition professionals therefore became less interested in the least-cost diet for workers and instead focused on the *best* diet for optimum public health.

To determine the ideal diet, experts measured vitality through a global comparison of bodies across eating cultures. Revelations about nutrition had come in the form of a new discovery: the vitamin, which experts found, through animal studies, made itself known through the measurable presence or absence of nutritional deficiencies in the body. The rise of the League of Nations post–WWI led to the rise in cross-national scientific collaborations, particularly the League of Nations Mixed Committee of Experts on Nutrition, an international research group of nutritionists.[44] The work of this committee measured the benefits of diet by measuring bodies, using this cross-national evidence to understand nutritional adequacy and deficiency.

The committee's widely discussed final report supported the superiority of the Northern European meat and dairy–centered diet.[45] Those cultures that were most similar to the American meat and dairy–centered diet were declared to be healthier. For example, the studies reported on the superior health of the African Maasai and the Indian Sikhs and attributed this to their consumption of milk.[46] Subsequent reanalysis of these studies has shown that their methodologies were faulty in the extreme. The researchers misrepresented their own fieldwork by underreporting the variety in the diet of the nearby vegetarian Kikiyu and by presenting the milk and meat-eating Maasai in a way that made the studies "propaganda pieces to show the deficiencies of vegetarianism [and] the benefits of milk."[47]

Conversely, cross-national comparisons of nutritional adequacy used the Asian body as a sign of nutritional, and political, deficiency. The vegetable-intensive Asian diet became representative of the colonized Asian nations.[48] Experts in the League of Nations and other studies used small Asian bodies as a sign of colonial subjugation and effeminacy. One of the most commonly cited studies at the time involved research in Bengal, India, where malnourishment due to a rice-only diet had led to the prevalence of the dietary deficiency disease, beri-beri.[49]

While these studies were epidemiological in nature, they were used in the popular press to explain the justice of colonizing these regions because the lack of meat-eating made them less aggressive. For example, an article in the *Saturday Evening Post*, "The Non-Beef-Eating Nations," described the Chinese as "peaceable and inoffensive as we would suppose a nation of rice-eaters might necessarily be" and "the rice-eating Hindoos at one time took a better position among the nations than they do now, but neither in war nor peace did they attain to anything of the standard of Europe or America."[50] The fact that the Russians and the Japanese (seldom cited as inferior rice-eaters in this rhetoric) had invaded large parts of China at the turn of the century reinforced the idea of the Chinese as not warlike. These peoples were seen as conquerable, defeated by diet. As noted earlier, union leaders took up ideas of the inferior Chinese diet to advocate an extension of the Chinese Exclusion Acts, because Chinese workers ostensibly accepted lower-wages due to the lower cost of their diet.

Western nutritionist accounts of the Chinese diet during this time period describe a population on the verge of mass starvation due to lack of vitamins and protein. Like meat, milk became a key food in this discourse. For example, USDA publicist T. Swann Harding argued in popular magazine articles that the Chinese diet was seriously deficient in protein: "The Chinese eat about one seventh as much meat as Americans. Milk is scarce in China and often viewed askance when available. It, therefore, appears that the Chinese have been consistently under-nourished since ancient days." To Harding, lack of milk and malnourishment went hand in hand, but even more interesting is the *use* to which Harding puts these superficial cross-national comparisons of diet, attributing dietary deficiency to a deficiency in national character: "Today, the Chinese is peaceful, sequacious, unprogressive, unenterprising, non-persevering; his stature is poor, his physique bad, his mortality high."[51] The idea that Asian bodies were enfeebled, due to lack of an adequate diet, justified imperial projects of colonization.[52]

Yet, instead of the struggle between reformers and the mass public over diet in the Gilded Age, the American public accepted the experts' claim that the American milk and meat diet represented a common source of national belonging: their shared identity as members of a powerful nation made strong by diet. As Helen Veit's history of World War I eating has shown, Americans united around Progressivism's "confidence in expertise, social-scientific knowledge, centralized administration, and the possibility of positive social change." This war-based unity made "food and its management patriotic projects and extending the state's reach into the home, onto dinner plates, and into kitchen cabinets." After decades of resistance to reformers seeking to discipline workers' eating habits, wartime unity convinced workers to embrace personal self-control over eating, making the war victory a "victory over ourselves."[53] This shared vision of national superiority also provided a tool for the working class to argue that they deserved more in their own society, especially once they became the soldiering bodies carrying out national military projects.

Nevertheless, the nutritionists' generalization of "just rice" as the common and universal Asian diet was simply incorrect. J. L. Buck, agronomist and the husband of writer Pearl Buck, studied the Chinese diet during the 1920s and '30s and found it to be adequate both in protein and calories.[54] In fact, food historians describe the Chinese as "among the best fed populations of Asia" for most of the last seven centuries. As a result, "the poor in China ate better in this respect than did the rich of Europe and, later, of America."[55] By 1900, "China was producing not only calories, but sufficient supplies of Vitamin A, Vitamin C, and other nutrients. The Chinese managed to produce vast quantities of vegetables, beans, and fish, pigs and chickens—enough to provide a basic living for all but the poorest."[56] Asian populations at the time, however, were experiencing waves of famine exacerbated by British colonial policy, leading to dietary deficiencies.[57]

The membership of the nutrition committee makes clear why all other diets fared badly compared to the milk-intensive diet. One of its main members was University of Wisconsin nutrition scientist E. V. McCollum, one of the early twentieth-century pioneer nutrition scientists whose animal feeding studies led to the discovery of the first vitamin: vitamin A. Like Atwater before him, he was also one of the premier purveyors of popular nutrition advice at the time, writing several books and over a hundred popular articles on the "New Nutrition." McCollum initiated the idea of "protective foods," particular foods that protect and maintain complete nutrition in a diet and therefore protect the body from nutrition deficiencies. McCollum's work emphasized milk as the ultimate "protective" food.

McCollum drew a direct parallel between milk-centered dietary practice and the success of Northern Europeans as a race. In his popular and widely read book, *The Newer Nutrition,* McCollum stated:

> The peoples who have made liberal use of milk as a food, have, in contrast [to non-milk-drinking peoples], attained greater size, greater longevity, and have been much more successful in the rearing of their young. They have been more aggressive than the non-milk using peoples, and have achieved much greater advancement in literature, science and art. They have developed in a higher degree educational and political systems which offer the greatest opportunity for the individual to develop his powers. Such development has a physiological basis, and there seems every reason to believe that it is fundamentally related to nutrition.[58]

He compares this superior diet to "[t]hose peoples who have employed the leaf of the plant as their sole protective food" who "are characterized by small stature, relatively short span of life, high infant mortality, and by contented adherence to the employment of the simple mechanical inventions of their forefathers."[59]

What cannot be ignored in these efforts is McCollum's close relationship with the dairy industry. He began his animal feeding experiments at the University of Wisconsin, the foremost dairy state of the period. It was during these experiments that he discovered that there was an undiscovered nutritional substance necessary to animal growth. McCollum isolated this substance, eventually called vitamin A, from dairy fat. The dairy industry trade journal, *Hoard's Dairymen,* and National Dairy Council publications quoted McCollum's findings widely, showing how various animals thrived on a milk diet and failed to thrive without. Concerned about the competition between butter and margarine—a nondairy product—*Hoard's* and other dairy industry media latched on to McCollum's vitamin study. *Hoard's* devoted a special issue to McCollum's work.[60]

McCollum sacralized the milk-intensive Yankee / Northern European diet in both his popular books and his nutrition policies. Milk became the "perfect" food.[61] The creation of dietary ideals—of one truly perfect food, or one truly perfect diet—placed one diet at the top and demoted the rest to less than ideal, even going so far as to denigrate particular diets—especially Chinese, African, and Indian vegetarian or low-meat diets—as debilitating.

Armed with the "fact" of American dietary superiority, social workers began to discourage new immigrants from continuing their ethnic food traditions and encourage an Americanization of their diet, whitening their meals with cream sauces and fresh milk as a beverage on the side. This early twentieth-century project of assimilation was also, sometimes explicitly but also by implication, a project of perfecting American society. A perfect, uniform American diet eaten by a nutritionally informed public would lead to perfect physical bodies and, particularly, healthy, well-adjusted schoolchildren who would become perfect citizens, more productive workers, and better soldiers.[62] As food historian Harvey Levenstein has argued, improved nutrition as a solution to the bodily impacts of economic inequality also depoliticized the physical impacts of inequality.[63] Perfect bodies became the way to display the perfection of the American social body, and to hide income disparities.

Ironically, McCollum was particularly aware of the benefits of vegetables, particularly leafy greens, knowledge he acquired through his animal feeding experiments. As he later describes in his *History of Nutrition,* he found in those experiments that ground-up leaves provided significant nutritional protection in animal feed. While nutritionists were not yet aware of all the chemistry involved in protective foods, the research of McCollum and others were beginning to show evidence of vitamins in foods other than milk. Yet, even before these discoveries, McCollum realized that leafy greens provided something that kept animals strong. He wrote an article in *McCall's* magazine, "Are You Eating the Protective Foods—Milk and Leaves?" that recognized the nutrition in both milk and greens.[64]

Yet, despite this recognition of both dairy and greens as nutritious, McCollum's primary focus in nutrition policy involved the promotion of milk. McCollum and others, such as USDA nutritionist Mary Swartz Rose, promoted dietary standards and improved nutrition at the USDA focused on the benefits of milk. Both McCollum and Rose were members of the Rockefeller-funded League of Nations Health Committee that wrote the cross-national study. It is therefore not surprising that the Maasai and the Sikh milk-based diet emerged as superior.

Why this lack of attention to vegetables, especially leafy greens? Of course, economic interests play a part in this explanation: there was no politically organized leafy green economic interest, while dairy interests were highly organized at the local, state, and national levels. In addition, before McCollum's discovery of vitamins in the 1910s, home economists and nutrition scientists did not recognize any nutrition benefit in vegetables. Instead, some were considered a "luxury"—salads and asparagus appear mostly in the "fancy" and "delicate" menus of cookbooks. "Salads were so strongly identified with the upper ranks of society," Laura Shapiro states, "the lady of the house was expected to make the salads herself" while not including salads in meals to servants, who got pickles instead.[65] What did not appear on these high-status tables were the dark leafy greens that characterized Asian, Southern, and African American diets. Nutrition advice therefore followed racial, ethnic, and sectional politics that sacralized the cream-based New England diet and treated other peoples' eating as degenerate and less civilized. The diets of marginal people must be inferior, according to this logic, because the people who ate them were subjugated. On the other hand, according to boosters of the Northern dairy diet, "A casual look at the races of people seems to show that those using much milk are the strongest physically and mentally, and the most enduring of the peoples of the world. Of all races, the Aryans seem to have been the heaviest drinkers of milk and the greatest users of butter and cheese, a fact that may in part account for the quick and high development of this division of human beings."[66]

Given the racial rhetoric of the day portraying the Chinese as effeminate and enfeebled, it is not surprising McCollum saw the Chinese "leaf" diet as a mark of degeneracy, drawing the parallel between gastropolitical racial exclusions and the politics of health and nutrition. In his analysis of anti-Chinese rhetoric, Gerald O'Brien illustrates how racial exclusions fit into common metaphors of society as a physical body: "Just as the integrity of our own bodies may be threatened by contaminating external elements, so too is the social body vulnerable to corruption by invading sub-groups." In anti-Chinese rhetoric of this period, the metaphor of "indigestibility" was commonly used to describe the inability of Asian groups to assimilate into American culture, as "peoples swallowed whole whom our digestive juices do not digest."[67] From this perspective, the idea of the ideal body politic and the ideal body were assumed to be congruent. In the body metaphor of society, ingestion represents belonging, digestibility represents assimilation, and inedibility becomes the metaphor for social exclusion.[68] Marginal groups, such as the leaf-eating Asians, considered improper eaters, were also indigestible as American citizens.

The northern areas of Yankee settlement were the major dairy regions of the country. Dairy interests in these states saw the link between celebrating the Yankee diet as creating a superior citizen and the creation of a prosperous agricultural economy based on a high-value commodity: milk. Milk was intertwined in a narrative of perfection that included pictures of pudgy babies with Anglo names advertising various milk formula products, as well as with school curricula that created the iconic acceptable child as one who was fully "American," that is, without signs of immigrant "old ways and a great drinker of milk." In this way, the Yankee dairy-intensive diet became a sign of ideal American citizenship.[69]

Making the Yankee diet the healthy way of eating created a purity politics that cleansed other racial, ethnic, and regional ways of eating from the idea of American citizenship. This political cleansing created a hygienic politics that promoted one way of eating as perfect and healthy and a world consisting of perfect and imperfect eaters. The result of purity politics was the exclusion of certain people and their ways of eating, making them lesser citizens in the American politic.

But, at the same time, the introduction of hygienic food practices also was powerful and life-saving. Purity made a difference for children drinking cows' milk, for survival in hospitals, and for extending urban life-spans. Yet, purification, as a symbol of citizenship and virtue, had disturbing results in the hands of American reformers. Eventually, the politics of purity created new problems, troublesome dilemmas that, today, defy resolution. Part II will describe how the hygienic politics of purity has become a conundrum, leading to "treadmills of purity" that exacerbate rather than resolve our current problems.

PART II

Ferment

5

Good Food, Bad Romance

JAMIE OLIVER IS CRYING AGAIN. He thought he could get the Huntington, Virginia, school lunch ladies "on his side." But they won't admit his food is better than the processed pre-packaged meals they defrost and serve to students. The children, it turns out, prefer the warmed-up pizza to his freshly baked chicken. Even the usual apples and bananas on the standard lunch food tray tend to end up in the garbage. Oliver cries a lot on his *Food Revolution* show. He has a mission: to bring good food to children in school cafeterias. In his TED talk he describes as his goal "to teach every child about food." So he picks himself up and tries again, because there is always another dinner and with this next one, he thinks, he can convince children to eat what he makes for them.

Oliver is just one of the many food activists seeking to change how children eat. They work by trying to change cafeteria food, to bring school gardens to campuses, and to teach children how to cook. They are striving to wrench children from the fast food that manages to fit eerily into national nutrition guidelines and, especially, school budgets. In the fight for the child's stomach, whole foods activists are winning skirmishes, but the industrial, processed food sector continues to be the overall victor. For, despite all this social action in favor of better diets, Americans aren't eating more fruits and vegetables. According to the Centers for Disease Control, the percentage of adults eating more than two fruit and three vegetables a day has been dropping.[1] Nearly every year, a new investigative committee comes out with a report that cites 30, soon to be 40, and eventually more than 50 percent of all American citizens are or will be overweight or obese. These reports say again and again that we need to change our nutrition advice strategies, yet all food advice still goes back to the "eat more vegetables" and "eat less carbs, fat, sugar" recommendation. "People have heard the advice to eat less and move more for years," a committee member of one of these reports noted, "and during that time a large number of Americans have become obese."[2]

Nutritionists call this high-fat, high-sugar, high-meat way of eating the "Standard American Diet" or S. A. D. The American diet is also S. A. D. because of what it is not: it is bereft of vegetables and low in whole grains and fiber. Nutritionists constantly cajole Americans to eat more vegetables and fiber, while food manufacturers are sneaking more fiber into processed foods. Globally, the move from the more common vegetable, fiber, and carbohydrate-intensive diet to this more American way of eating is often referred to as "the nutrition transition." Nutritionists have observed the globalization of this dietary transition: carbohydrates go from complex to simple; meat becomes the center of the meal; more calories come from fat; people walk less and drive more.[3] Research shows the results of these new habits: greater heart disease, climbing obesity rates, especially for children, and an increase in diabetes, to mention just a few of the health problems.[4] Nutrition researchers like Barry Popkin have documented the expansion of the S. A. D. throughout the world, a phenomenon he describes as a "global pandemic."[5]

This story of American colonization of the global stomach parallels other American cultural invasions. In the global media, the fat American body represents this diet of "bad" choices. For many across the world, the American citizen, once considered the model of Enlightenment democracy, has become an icon of a degenerate, *Jersey Shore* lifestyle of bad choices, a symbol for the larger global-gluttonous-degenerate American juggernaut of military expansion, carbon emissions, and the widening Global Waistline. Social theorist Jean Baudrillard describes America as the "original version of modernity."[6] S. A. D. has become a symbol of how that modernity has deceived us, standing not for the Progressive promise of healthy prosperity, but for a dystopic, degraded, unsustainable future, spreading McDonald's and KFCs across the globe as symbols of the growing world health and environmental crises.

Where did S. A. D. come from? Some, like Michael Pollan, Eric Schlosser, and Mark Bittman, argue that this massive transition in consumption originates in the industrialization of agricultural production, which led to diets dominated by processed food and factory-farmed meat that are filled with artificial flavors to trick the taste buds.[7] Food policy researchers Tim Lang and Michael Heasman describe this transition to processed food diets as "a period of unprecedented and rapid change in the food system,"[8] through food chain integration and control systems that have led to "astonishing leaps in productivity," as well as a doubling of economic concentration in US food manufacturing so that "100 firms now account for 80 percent of all value-added in the sector."[9] The beef-processing sector has become so industrialized that four processing firms now control over 80 percent of the industry.

The new fast meat system was not just a technical transition. The new organization of intensive meat processing required breaking the traditionally strong meatpacking unions. Fast meat now relies primarily on immigrant, often undocumented, workers. And this transition happened in parallel with the rise of new food reform movements: Slow Food, organic food, and other alternative food systems. "Ironically," Ted Genoways notes, "at the very moment that enlightened eaters were growing obsessed by the idea of 'slow food,' the meat industry was becoming overwhelmingly staffed by recent immigrants—many without legal employment status—as a way of pushing production lines to go faster and faster."[10] The "food revolution" described by so many food reformers was, in fact, a partition of the food system into two distinct systems: one determined by increasing speed and decreasing cost and a separate quality-based system that, by comparison, requires more time, labor, and materials. Not surprisingly, then, nutritionists, using an index of healthy eating (more fruits and vegetables, fewer trans-fats and salt), found that the gap in healthy eating scores is widening between rich and poor. As cheap food becomes even more industrialized and processed, the poor are eating more of it while those who have the means avoid it. The poor are then blamed for their faulty lifestyles, leading to new policies to control the consumption of those at fault. In fact, commenting on the widening healthy food gap study, nutritionists recommended that food stamp programs "restrict benefits to more healthful foods, as has been done by the Special Supplemental Nutrition Program for Women, Infants and Children (WIC)."[11]

Part I of this book described four historical eras, showing how eating in each of those eras mirrored the American culture of the time: the tensions, hopes, fears and divisions, the exclusions, inequalities, and power relations. Any explanation of our current eating issues, and attempts to change American eating, must draw on this history. Any explanation of our current concerns needs to consider how previous efforts at changing eating existed in a historical American struggle between self-discipline and self-indulgence that made cheap food—in particular cheap meat—the center of the American plate. Michael Pollan and others have argued that cheap food is simply a way for the overheated industrial system to get rid of its surplus. Yet, cheap food solves other social problems as well: the tensions between and among various groups in American society, the struggle over good wages and who gets those wages, the struggle over what those wages can pay for, especially meat—all fed the growth of the industrial system that made meat cheaper. This gothic horror of industrialized meat—the Confined Animal Feeding Operations that turn sentient beings into meat-making machines, the slaughterhouses filled with undocumented workers who accept employment there at the risk of life and limb, the American populace becoming a public health scare—grew out of the cheap food solution.

Understanding S. A. D. also requires knowing the ways in which the cheap meat-centered diet stigmatized fiber-filled diets of other Americans— the greens and beans eating cultures of China, Mexico, and the black and white South. Instead, less meat-intensive, yet no less American, cuisines transformed into a meat-centered plate. The traditional Southern "three-veg" meal became the box of fried chicken; Chinese takeout became primarily meat and rice with vegetables as flavoring; the bean and corn–centered Mexican cuisine became a corn or wheat tortilla as container for the mostly meaty substance inside. In other words, cheap food is not just a capitalist conspiracy; it is a class bargain fed by public consent. Cheap food fits into a larger American bargain among industry (cheap wages), workers (cheap food), and the middle class (moral superiority), enabling each to fill a role and to gain advantages from that role.

THE ROMANTIC MORALITY PLAY OF FOOD

Like their nineteenth-century forebears, today's food reform movements are romantic, emphasizing the transformation of personal habits as the road to social change. And like the Romantic reformers of the American antebellum period, good eating habits and healthy lifestyles present an opportunity to demonstrate middle-class moral superiority and to legitimize the middle class as the providers of moral uplift to other members of society. Just as Sylvester Graham blamed human "sensual excesses" for the rise of epidemics,[12] reformers blame Americans' personal eating habits, their inability to resist temptation, for the rise of the industrial food system. Reformers didactically exhort Americans to return to civic republican self-discipline and Yankee morality as the way out of large problems such as climate change: "If every U. S. citizen ate just one meal a week (any meal) composed of locally and organically raised meats and produce," state Barbara Kingsolver et al. in

Animal, Vegetable, Miracle, "we would reduce our country's oil consumption by over 1.1 million barrels of oil every week. . . . Small changes in buying habits can make a big difference."[13] "You can argue," they state, "that our wishes don't count, but humans are good at making our dreams manifest."[14] Reformers see changing the behavior of others as a cure for the ills of industrial agriculture: "The deceptively simply act of eating fresh, seasonal foods grown close to home is creating a wave of change," states Amy Cotler in her book, *The Locavore Way.* "It moves us away from the horrors of industrial farms and feedlots."[15]

In other words, today's food reformers are fulfilling the traditional American middle-class role by turning to a civic republican purification of personal lifestyle as the solution to social problems. The moral answer to the question "How do we change the world?" is, once again, "We must change ourselves." Those who do not participate in personal change are then deemed unworthy. Romance is embedded, once again, in a troublesome politics of purity that makes romantic visions of ideal diets the solution to larger, more complex social problems. This dietary reform conversation, once again, turns larger questions of social and political inequality into a problem of self-discipline.

And, once again, these purported solutions do not work. Like the nineteenth-century reformers, today's food activists exhort us to make and eat home-cooked meals, yet families increasingly eat the fast and cheap food prepared by others, either commercially prepared convenience foods or away from home. Away-from-home eating doubled between 1960 and 2000, according to the National Health Interview Survey. The authors of the survey, Ashima Kant and Barry Graubard, describe the trend this way: "driven by rising incomes, two-income households, and demand for convenience, this period has seen an unprecedented growth in the number of commercial food establishments, with an especially dramatic growth of the fast-food industry."[16] In other words, S. A. D. productively resolved another American tension: the struggle over which full-time parent worker would cook the evening meal. Food reformers continue to tell Americans that they should resist these trends, to eat at home, cook from scratch, eat together and eat locally, without recognizing the broader reasons people live the lifestyle they criticize. Convenience food, like cheap food, is a bargain that solves the tension between women who want to work outside the home and men who don't want to cook inside it.

Like past counterparts, food reformers fill the pages of the popular press, using themselves as examples, writing about their lifestyle changes, and inviting others to join in. Using their own experiences of purification, they try to change the consciousness of others and move them toward their life-style as the right one: "bringing good food to others."[17] Reform once again becomes didactic, about teaching others the right way to live or, as Barbara Kingsolver puts it, "We'd surely do better, if only we *knew* any better." The problem is the ignorant consumer who, according to Wendell Berry, simply "no longer knows or imagines the connections between eating and the land, and is therefore necessarily passive and uncritical—in short, a victim. When food, in the minds of eaters, is no longer associated with farming and with the land, then the eaters are suffering a kind of cultural amnesia that is misleading and dangerous."[18] Like Sylvester Graham exhorting women to bake their own bread, today's food reformers believe that change will come when they convince consumers to "know your food," or even better to grow and cook their own food. This "if they only knew" approach to food system change assumes that change is a matter of others learning the truth about "where their food comes from." The movie *Food, Inc.* represents that kind of contemporary reform didacticism: it lifts the veil of the commercial food media to show the true essence of industrial agricultural production, in hopes that this information "would necessarily trigger a desire for local, organic food and people would be willing to pay for it."[19]

But, once again, like the century before, defining "good food" has become a process of defining a romantic ideal, an escape from the current industrial agricultural production system by a leap to the outside, the alternative: organic standards, fair trade, local food systems. Yet, even more so than in the past, food reformers seek to change the system by putting a boundary between nature and culture, purity and danger, and thereby escaping from culture and danger into an ideal world of nature and purity, a perfect world that does not exist. *Food, Inc.*, for example, begins by showing how the industrial food system presents a romantic view of food production on its packaging. The heroic farm family, in the green meadow, with the grazing animals and the pristine crop, represents an ideal of purity. The movie promises to unveil the romance, to show the reality beneath. But the notion of unveiling is itself romantic, a promise that the "real" good food can be found underneath the veil.

Yet, the search for purity, for cleanliness, for escape from society, is a dream, and dreams are something our commercial-industrial system is willing to provide. It incorporates—co-opts—these romances into new forms of profit—brands—to sell to us to save us from ourselves, to sell us the Right

Way to Live (when they aren't selling us the comfort of Eat What You Want). Sincere social activists create new alternative worlds—inspired by the old romances of revelation, nature, and Europe, adding a nostalgia for old ways of life—only to find that these get taken up as new commercial brands.

THE NEW EUROPEAN ROMANCE

The Mediterranean Diet and Slow Food both exhibit all the telltale signs of nineteenth-century civic romanticism: nature, Europe, and revelation. Current food reformer Alice Waters represents this triple embrace: often described as a visionary, with roots in European cooking and faithful to nature. Like visionaries of the American past, she consistently describes her experience in Europe as an "awakening": "It was really an awakening for me," she says of her first visit to a Paris. "I felt like I had never really eaten before. I had liked certain things but I didn't understand how it fit into people's lives in a delicious way. When I went [to Paris] and walked past the markets and ate in the little restaurants, it was like a revelation. . . . So when I came home, I felt like I could really make this happen in my own life."[20] Michael Pollan tells a somewhat different, and more masculine, awakening story in *The Omnivore's Dilemma,* starting his book with a fast-food hamburger and ending it in an epic hunt of a wild pig, a transcendentalist meeting with nature, accompanied by a European sidekick.

Slow Food movement members also tell the romantic story of nature, Europe, and revelation, with a didactic mission to educate others. They congregate in "convivia" where they cook, eat, and talk about reeducating Americans to European slow eating and tasting: "I think that's one of the big things about Slow Food, taste education. We as a country really have developed this taste for fat," one member at a local California convivium opined to sociologist Sarita Gaytan. "I think you just have to win people over with taste and convince them to slow down and enjoy life a little bit. The Italians, they have eating down right."[21] Another convivium member narrated his awakening: "So when I went to France and went into a cheese store, I think I fainted. I mean, I had no idea there were so many varieties of cheese, each one better than another, in one space in the world."[22] Slow Food convivia members narrate stories of awakening to a healthier European food culture as a mode of escape from American industrial food and the obesity epidemic. Their goal is to get away from the American way of life by eating unlike

Americans. Convivium leader and Slow Food activist Deborah Madison writes that Slow Food is also less American because it is more in line with nature, in that members are "seeking a tempo of life that is more in step with life's natural rhythms, unlike America's present fast-paced model."[23]

This love of Europe brings food reformers together with more popular diet writers who sacralize Europe as a place of thin bodies. In particular, the French appear to have their own "dietary paradox" that enables them to be modern, Western, and healthy, while eating good food. A popular diet book of the 2000s, *French Women Don't Get Fat*, publicized itself in the classic way as a "non-diet" book that enabled eaters to enjoy food without consequence, through, once again, an awakening to a "radical change in how you think and live."[24]

In this celebration of European lifestyles, the Mediterranean Diet reigns supreme. Typical of American media coverage, Robin Roberts of *Good Morning America* moderated a segment entitled "World's Healthiest Diet: What's the Mediterranean Secret?" She introduces *Good Morning America* medical contributor Dr. Marie Savard, a wispily thin, 60-something blond woman, discussing a study of the eating habits of 23,000 Greek men and women participating in the European Prospective Investigation into Cancer and Nutrition (EPIC). Asked to comment, Dr. Savard states enthusiastically: "I really think the Mediterranean Diet is the Holy Grail of Diets. It's the one that we are looking for. It improves survival, no question. It lowers the risk of diabetes, heart disease, even cancers."[25] Savard is not the only nutritionist to embrace the Mediterranean Diet as saving Americans from themselves. Many others also focus on the Mediterranean Diet and how it keeps Europeans thin and "heart-healthy," while S. A. D. explains why Americans are so fat and prone to heart attacks. Nutritionists embrace Mediterranean eaters as that part of the industrialized West that escaped the nutrition transition.[26]

Yet, the accompanying article on the study discussed by Savard, on the *ABCnews* website, did not make the same claims about this way of eating. While calling the Mediterranean Diet "the poster child for healthy eating," the article quotes experts like Dr. David Katz, director of the Prevention Research Center at Yale University School of Medicine in New Haven, Connecticut, who states: "Once you have a mostly plant-based diet and eat few processed foods, almost any variation on the theme will be fine."[27]

Plant-based diets with few processed foods characterize the vast majority of world diets throughout history. In fact, it characterizes many of the ethnic cultures whose diets have been systematically stigmatized in American nutrition history: the Asian diet's emphasis on vegetables, the Southern / Soul meat-and-three-veg diet, the Mexican corn-rice-and-bean-centered meal. But, instead of rethinking the historical stigmatization of these diets, Americans are sold on the idea that the one perfect way of eating is intrinsically European.[28] The Mediterranean Diet is no longer just an eating practice or a set of nutrition guidelines, it has become its own American dietary moral reform vision. For Americans, a thin, long, mentally and physically sensual healthy life is found in Europe.

How did the Mediterranean Diet achieve this sacred status among American nutritionists? The answer to that question starts with Ancel Keys, the creator of the K ration during WWII, and the principal investigator in the Minnesota Semi-Starvation experiments, who in the 1950s discovered the relationship between types of diet and the prevalence of heart disease through a collaborative study with European scientists called the Seven Country Study. This study became famous as the first to announce the dangers of a high cholesterol diet.

Yet, it was not until the '70s that Keys began to promote the Mediterranean Diet as the solution to American dietary problems. In the first edition of their popular book on the topic, *Eat Well and Stay Well,* Keys and his co-author wife did not associate the low cholesterol diet with Mediterranean cuisine. There aren't even very many "Italian" dishes in that first edition from 1959. Most recipes in the book are for American dishes with somewhat less saturated fat or cholesterol-containing ingredients. There is none of the typical celebration of Mediterranean-ness in either food practices or healthy lifestyle. It was only with the 1975 edition, renamed *How to Eat Well and Stay Well the Mediterranean Way,* that the evocation of this region became part of the salvation of the fat American body.[29] According to one Keys's biography, the nutrition scientist was greatly inspired, originally, by his long sojourns in Italy and by his childhood in the East Bay of California.[30] California cuisine has always included more fresh food, and the rise of the California fresh fruit and vegetable industry is part and parcel of a food regime that favors California's Mediterranean agroecology.

The highbrow American media has also embraced the Mediterranean Diet. Food writers celebrate European eating as part of a rich and fulfilling way of life. *New York Times* food writer Frank Bruni, for example, celebrates pork while placing "pig heaven" in Italy and not in the American South, replaying the sectionalist bias against Southern ways of life. Another *New*

York Times food columnist, Martha Rose Shulman, has a very well-known cookbook, *Mediterranean Harvest: Vegetarian Recipes for the World's Healthiest Cuisine.* Recently, she did an excellent series on a traditional American food, collard greens. However, she began the column not with the usual celebration of the region where the dish comes from—the American South—but with a remark about her lifelong distaste for the traditional way of cooking it. Southern pork is not heavenly enough and its traditional greens are not the European version.[31]

Ironically, as many Americans extol the Mediterranean Diet, Europeans, as well as the rest of the world, are making the transition to American eating, the S. A. D. diet, becoming obese and prone to the diseases of affluence they had until now managed to avoid. Recent studies of the rise in obesity among Mediterranean children indicate that the dietary transition is catching up with Europe. And, despite the portrayal of Europeans as instilled with the idea of food as pleasure, food anxiety is not entirely absent from European bookstore shelves. As *Le Monde* put it, "La France" is "sur le voie des Etats-Unis" (on the American path—that is, French women *do* get fat).[32] If the French continue on this path, the Americanization of their diet will catch them up—obesity-wise—with Americans by 2020.[33]

Europeans, for their part, fight guerilla battles against the American stomach by embracing the vestiges of their own traditional cultures and their rural countrysides. Europe, one of most densely urbanized regions of the world, protects its stomach from America by turning to its own rural traditional cultures.[34] The icon representing American influence is the Monster of McDonald's, which has invaded the European town square (including, most recently, the Louvre). Resistance to American eating practices and American globalization has become increasingly interconnected, with McDonald's the iconic crossroads between the two. Both Slow Food's Carlo Petrini and the alter-globalization movement's Jose Bove target McDonald's as their focus of resistance to, in tandem, globalization and *malbouffe* (junk food).

In the food movement, the romantic re-embrace of nature often involves a re-embrace of the past, a rediscovery of "where our food comes from." This narrative tells a story about how we have become separated from our food and how eating locally, or rediscovering the system that grows our food, will repair our bodies and help change the food system. The bad quality of food comes from our separation from food production, which is a product of the industrialization of food. By getting closer to our food, we can repair our relationship with it and thereby overcome our broken system. Yet, ironically, the path to becoming "close to nature" lies across the sea, in European cuisine.

Sacralizations always have their ironies, and there are several ironies with the idea of the Mediterranean Diet as the perfect diet and with the European Slow Food movement as the politics of resistance to the global American juggernaut. First, the Mediterranean peasant class that is the purported source of this dietary lifestyle has basically ceased to exist. Mediterranean rural regions have experienced a rapid decline in peasant populations at the same time that they have increased their leisure-seeking and—substantially British—retirement populations in recent years.[35] Those empty farmhouses discovered and restored by American women recovering from romantic breakups are empty for a reason: the loss of rural economies and their working agricultural landscapes in these regions. Yet, urban Europeans look to their rapidly disappearing peasant countryside cultures to save their bodies from the American diet. Therefore, Slow Food is one of those movements to revive a way of life after it has gone.

Secondly, the Mediterranean Diet is also a relatively mythical food practice, in that most Europeans do not eat strictly in this manner today, nor have they ever. Food studies scholar Janet Chrzan dubs this sacralization of Tuscany and the Mediterranean Diet "the Tuscan Myth." "Tuscan food is considered to embody the health-giving principles of the Mediterranean Diet and, thus," she states, "adoption of Tuscan food-habits is a powerful means to transform the self into a more healthful cultural and biological agent." The Mediterranean Diet is a kind of "idealized embodiment" of "beliefs and behaviours surrounding a mythologised Mediterranean diet." Chrzan argues that these ideals are class-based and represent "deep reservations about present American cultural, familial, and nutritional realities." According to the Americans she interviewed, Tuscan food is simple, fresh, and pure, a "projected purity" that is "reflective of American patterns of belief more than Tuscan food habits."[36]

Graham Robb paints a more realistic story of Mediterranean food history in his book *The Discovery of France,* which, unlike the slew of current cookbooks on the diet, never dented the top 100 US bestsellers. Robb describes how French peasants historically had to sleep through much of the winter because they did not have enough available calories to get them through that season moving and awake. Historically, *simple* peasant food, in Mediterranean France, was often *not enough.*[37] In fact, as food scholar Rachel Laudan describes in her work on Slow Food, the pasta-centric diet of Italy was never possible before WWII, because Italy was never able to produce enough wheat for this kind of diet.[38] Chrzan says of Tuscany: "Until recently the region was legendary for its poverty."

This is not to say that the S. A. D. is, in fact, a good diet, and that the Mediterranean Diet is, in fact, a bad diet. This is also not to say that Alice Waters's food isn't great, which it is; or that Pollan's exhortations to "Eat real food, mostly plants" isn't excellent advice. S. A. D. is clearly a source of health problems, but sacralizing Europe and certain eating practices over other equally healthy practices is also a problem. My question, instead, is this: why is Europe presented as the only source of good food and "the good life"? Why not Japanese or Chinese diets, equally low in saturated fat and high in fiber? What about African American Soul and Southern country cooking meat-and-three-veg diets that are filled with beans and leaves? Why not the bean-and-corn-centered Mexican cuisine? Couldn't these be candidates to save Americans from their obesogenic plight? Aren't most diets in relatively temperate parts of the world essentially the fiber-filled, low sugar, low fat, less meat diets that are counter to S. A. D.?

Despite the universality of dietary balance in most cuisines, localist and Slow Food movement actors get caught up in the Mediterranean narrative, which links good food with European sacralization of either peasant rustic or aristocratic, highbrow ways of life. The US alternative food movement, especially Slow Food, is constantly accused of hypocrisy, with media accounts often noting "the perception that Slow Food is elitist and inaccessible to many people."[39] In a magazine article, Alice Waters, one of the mainstays of Slow Food USA, is reported to have "bristled" when a reporter broached this topic.[40] Yet, even the most sympathetic foodies agree that there is a disconnect between Slow Food USA and mainstream USA eaters, although, for the most part, they see mainstream lifestyle and processed food advertising as the source of the problem.

Whether or not the local, organic, and Slow Food movement is elitist, the gastro-tourism industry does not hesitate to translate Slow Food ideas into the commercial American culture of comfort, aristocratic distinction, commercial brands, and economic profit. Nowhere is this more obvious than in the food media. In particular, the Italian aspect of Slow Food gets sanctified in the pages of that paragon of middle-class food anxiety, the *New York Times,* which evokes Slow Food in various gastro-touristic travel articles, in ways never claimed by the founder of the Slow Food movement, Carlos Petrini. For example, *Philadelphia Inquirer* writer Frank Fitzpatrick uses Slow Food to sell Turin gastro-tourism in an article titled "Medal-worthy Food: Slowing Down in Tasty Turin." He describes a conversation with "the 31-year-old founder of the nation's hottest new gelateria," a man who is part of the new, entrepreneurial chef elite, a kind of Donald Trump version of the restauranteur. Article after article on these new entrepreneur chefs evokes Slow Food, Waters, and Petrini, draining them of their larger political ideals for the sake of selling a touristic story.

Troublesome but inevitable contradictions float to the surface as Waters and Slow Food get covered in the gastro-media—especially the *New York Times* food and travel sections. According to one article, Waters's simple cuisine signals that "[t]he idea of gastronomy would never again depend on preparations named for dead French nobles"; however, the same article ends with a description of Waters cooking for "bigwigs" in an Italian castle. Some articles on the food movement specifically celebrate the idea of Waters as a Francophile. Others flirt surprisingly often with symbols of regality. In one, a Turin star chef-entrepreneur type sniffs the air and states approvingly: "You can smell a city that has had a king" in reference to "those tasty traditions aristocrats engendered." Pleasure and taste is temptingly relinked to aristocracy. In another, the royalty is Prince Charles himself, promoting his new line of organic food, an article that describes Waters as "smitten" with the prince. While the movement espouses simple food and the simple life, others adorn the idea of Slow Food and standard-bearer Waters with symbols that evoke these royal roots.[41] This fetishization of a social movement for the sake of the tourist sector does not do the movement any good. It takes a healthy eating movement and sells it to the elite, further strengthening the link between privilege and healthy eating.[42] Commercial media and food companies then cater to the status-seeking motivations of the middle class by presenting processed soups, salad dressings, and other foods as "Tuscan."

Placed within the Europhilic–Europhobic context of American politics, the Mediterranean Diet and Slow Food are taken up by a media that caters to a distinction-seeking audience, as a status-claiming gourmet practice, and as a result, as a target of populist scorn. Every attempt to get people to eat better becomes a performance of Europhilic status-competition. The chapters of Pollan's *The Omnivore's Dilemma* tell this story perfectly: a brilliant beginning on the problems of a corn-based food economy veers into a description of organic agriculture as libertarian populist utopia, and finally devolves into a final chapter in which Pollan performs his own personal status sacralization ritual, pig hunting with an Italian advisor. In this chapter, Pollan combines

Transcendentalist love of nature and Jacksonian frontier independence (hunt your own) with a Europhilic love of artisanship (with an expert Italian huntsman who can prepare the pig beautifully). The result is author as icon, in this case an icon for both sides of the Europhilic–Europhobic coin.[43]

Looking at quality food as a romance is not a critique of quality itself. Protective boundaries to preserve quality are an important tool. Romance has always been a commercially successful story, whether it is the pulp romances of True Love or the romance of idealistic visions of social change. But, boundaries based on the romantic notions of essence and purity lead to confoundings, struggles to make distinctions between things that are intrinsically indistinct. Boundaries create social distinctions in status as well, meaning that romantic ideals tend to justify inequalities. For the middle classes, ideas about good food and purity become part of their moral culture of deservedness. Since the Gilded Age, the commercial media has known how to take those desires and turn them into desirable commercial products. One result is a rampage of money-making by actors at the edge of the movement culling some good ideas for simple profit while ignoring the larger message.

For, what is the Standard American Diet? "American" can mean the Western and industrialized, global mass production, big profit, cheap calorie system that, in fact, many consumers see as their way to save money for other things besides fueling their bodies. Or, American can mean what people in this country have traditionally eaten, our own homegrown diets, what our grandmothers ate, as Michael Pollan puts it. But who is "our" grandmother? There have been many grandmothers in this country and they have eaten different things in the country's history. If Americans do turn to an intrinsically American diet, what will they turn to?

This is an important question if we see food, as Part I of this book has shown, as intrinsically related to larger American ideas about freedom, order, identity, and, especially, morality. To say that American food is intrinsically bad says something about Americans in general. It's one thing to have snobbish Europeans denigrate the American diet. It's another thing to have the country's own nutritionists and media tell us that what Americans eat is basically unredeemable and that any attempt to improve eating requires discarding our own eating and, therefore, who we are. Rather than trying to escape ourselves, another possibility is to look within.

6

The Trouble with Purity

IN HIS ESSAY "THE TROUBLE WITH WILDERNESS," William Cronon gives us a different idea of wilderness, not as untouched nature "out there" but as an American idea, "a mirror" in which "we see the reflections of our own unexamined longing and desires." "For Americans," he states, "wilderness stands as the last remaining place where civilization, that all too human disease, has not fully infected the earth. It is an island in the polluted sea of urban-industrial modernity, the one place we can turn for escape from our own too-muchness." Cronon's now famous essay challenged the American idea of a world bifurcated between culture and the romantic view of wilderness as threatened by the contagion of civilization, of a world where nature represents freedom from the "too-muchness" of modern society.[1]

But, if the nature outside becomes a mirror of people's "longings and desires," doesn't the nature within do the same thing? Don't people's attempts to purify their own diets, to make their insides clean and to only eat food that is "natural," apart from modernity, replicate these bifurcations and boundaries between nature and culture? These questions are important not just in the realm of food politics but for the larger question of how people choose a sustainable future. How do people make sustainable change without falling into the bifurcated politics of purity or romance?

This question is particularly important today, when some people argue that, to adapt to the Anthropocene—that is, a world increasingly dominated by human intervention—we must embrace the synthetic to save nature through advanced technological systems: vat meat, hyperindustrialized vertical greenhouses, nuclear energy, and vast genetic modifications. Members of the Breakthrough project proclaim "The End of Environmentalism" and a "transcending of nature-based politics" to rescue the world through an accelerated transition to high technology.[2] Of course, this is just another romance of political bifurcation, a way to change the world that rejects the natural and embraces the synthetic.

Rather than seeing the world as separated by the boundaries of pure and dangerous, nature and culture, natural and synthetic, what if we just admit that such opposing categories have become a conundrum: an impossible struggle to split the world in two—a purified inside protected against a dangerous outside? Why not look at struggles over food purity as a story about these wider choices, where the mouth represents that boundary of contention, that place where we ask not "what should we eat?" but "*how* do we decide what to eat?" In other words, rather than seeing the solution as a search for the "real" boundary between nature and culture, why not see our current challenges as an opportunity for carrying out the tricky and painful political work necessary to decide where boundaries are set? In this chapter, we will begin by looking at how Americans continue to be trapped in a purity politics that has led to personal and national conundrums. The first two case studies are at different scales, showing how the bifurcated politics of purity affects both personal practices and national governance. Personal detoxification practices and the Food Safety Modernization Act are examples of these purity conundrums.

We will then look at one small but important exception, one that represents not an attempt to discover the true, natural boundary between organic and synthetic, but a political process that starts from the position that this boundary, not discoverable in nature, is constructed through a discursive political process: the decision-making processes of the National Organic Standards Board.

"Boundary-work" is an idea first used by sociologist Thomas Gieryn to describe the ways in which scientists separate science from nonscience. Studying how scientists present themselves as separate from the world, Gieryn has found that "attempts to demarcate science have failed": when you look closely at how scientists create boundaries between scientific ways of knowing and other ways, what you find is that the boundary is fuzzy and uncertain.[3] In fact, what Gieryn found was that scientists preserve their authority through the ideological boundaries of symbolism and metaphor, rather than through the tools of scientific objectivity—empiricism and falsifiability—that separate the "out there" from society. The Progressive Era diet ideologues, with their heavy reliance on metaphors of perfection and purity, are an example of how science and moral mission have mixed together in American dietary policy.

"Boundary" has functioned as a major metaphor in scientific ideas about diet. Sociologists Michele Lamont and Virag Molnar see boundary-work as both symbolic and social. They define "symbolic boundaries" as "conceptual distinctions made by social actors to categorize objects, people, practices, and even time and space. They are tools by which individuals and groups struggle over and come to agree upon definitions of reality." Social boundaries, on the other hand, are "objectified forms of social differences manifested in unequal access to and unequal distribution of resources (material and nonmaterial) and social opportunities." Groups seeking to achieve and maintain a higher social status, as well as greater access to resources and authority, autonomy, and privilege, use symbolic boundary-work to maintain social boundaries.[4] Pierre Bourdieu's study of "distinction" is an in-depth analysis of how classes use boundary-work to maintain separateness and achieve status.[5] In other words, once the symbolic boundaries become set as reality, as natural, they are used by some to gain power over others. The pure and sanitary food policies of the Progressive Era described in Part I were clearly an example of this form of symbolic politics, using ethnic and genetic ideals of purity as ways for particular groups to gain and maintain their social status.

Yet, purity politics also has material effects, ones not often described in studies of boundary-work, and some of which are beneficial. Without the sanitary protections put in place through Progressive policies, urban modern life would not have been possible, since cities require sanitary regulations to maintain population that would otherwise be overly vulnerable to epidemic diseases.[6] Sanitation, therefore, is a third kind of material boundary-work not commonly considered in the sociological discussions of boundaries. Because the growth of cities required sanitation, the relationship between symbolic and material boundaries has been a long-standing discussion in urban environmental history. Historians such as William Cronon have emphasized the symbolic aspects of modern ideas about nature as "wilderness" untouched by human hands. Urban environmental historians, however, have been faced with the need to explain the relationship between material forms of boundary-making that enabled people to live together in dense environments without being subjected to continual epidemics. Urban environmental historians Martin Mellosi and Joel Tarr argue that the rise of cities would not have been possible without significant boundary-work separating out—materially—clean from unclean. They show how epidemics hampered the growth of cities until sanitary systems—waterworks and waste removal, for example—were put into place.[7]

Food is another area where the symbolic work around boundaries becomes material. Large-scale food systems necessary to feed urban populations would not have been possible without food purity and safety regulations, that is, a material form of boundary-work.[8] Yet, as Part I showed, these necessary boundaries also became symbolic boundaries, creating social inequalities as some groups claimed greater purity and cleanliness.

Today the material boundary-work between clean and unclean eating, safe and unsafe food, has become problematic. One strategy has been to set up systems to protect humans from the minutest hint of dirt or germ. The first case study will show how the politics of purity affects personal ideas about good lifestyles, creating a middle-class romantic politics of "clean eating" dominated by notions of internal cleanliness as the "final frontier" in an endless process of hyper-purification I call the "treadmill of purity." The second case study expands these ideas to the national scale, through a look at the Food Safety Modernization Act. To implement this legislation, the FDA has proposed rules that ostensibly keep dangerous bacteria such as *Listeria* and *E. coli* O57:H7 out of produce. Yet, the rules impose significant expenses on farms and processors, and only larger industrial food producers have the resources to meet these rules. Examining the last few years of food scares, however, shows that large-scale foodborne illness problems are primarily a product of the same industrial food system that will be strengthened by this regulation. The legislation, and the FDA, have created a rule that makes a strong separation between food and nature. This hyper-purification creates a treadmill of purity on a national scale. The treadmill of purity describes the continual attempts to strengthen and re-strengthen the necessary but imperfect boundaries between purity and danger to the nth degree of perfect purity.

On the other hand, the decision-making process of the National Organic Standards Board (NOSB)—the third case study described here—represents another, less common, and less romantic form of food boundary-making that escapes the treadmill of purity. The NOSB is a deliberative advisory body that determines what ingredients should be allowed in organic food. For this reason, NOSB discussions and hearings provide an excellent window through which to view an alternative to the treadmill of purity. In its decision making over what to allow in organic food, the NOSB has created discursive boundaries—created through discussion—while admitting that true, ideal boundaries do not exist. The NOSB process has been a continually contested but remarkably successful discursive governance process by which members of a community decide what is "allowable" and "not allowable" in food certified as organic.

Ideals of good food have been caught in unrealistic and unattainable ideals of purity. These ideals are a trap in which people attempt to eliminate risk by reintensifying purification, only to lead to more problems, which lead to more intensive attempts at purification. These treadmills become a constant churning of anxiety about risk and attempts at purification that, in some cases, might actually increase risk. Only a less perfect, more open, and discursive kind of food boundary-work can keep American eaters "safe," if imperfectly so. As the final case study demonstrates, NOSB boundary-work, based on a discursive form of governance, represents a less perfect, but more effective, process.

CLEAN INSIDE AND OUT

In their movie *Food Matters,* James Colquhoun and Laurentine ten Bosch present detoxification as an escape from the pharmaceutical world of conventional medicine. Detoxification can mean many things, from simply avoiding sugar and alcohol for a period of time to more radical purges. In the movie and accompanying website videos, Colquhoun and ten Bosch invite the audience to detox with them: "We clean our body every day, taking a shower, but do we clean our insides? Do we think about that?" ten Bosch asks. "Animals in nature have this innate intelligence to go off feed, or fast, or restrict the food they eat when they are not feeling well," co-director James Colquhoun adds, using ideas of untouched nature to justify a three-day purge limiting food to green juices and salads.

The symbolic politics of pure insides has been a theme of American life since the abolitionist vegetarians of Fruitlands, who made manifest their ideas of a virtuous life by entering the gates of self-denial. By the Gilded Age, ideas about internal cleanliness had become a middle-class anxiety about the consequences of overindulgence. Laxative manufacturers advertised that their products enabled consumers to "eat what you want" without worrying about internal impurities. In the twentieth century, pharmaceutical companies sold products that promised internal cleanliness (fig. 6). The contaminant in today's discussion of detoxification is more likely to be our modern industrial system itself—pollutants in our food, air, and other products that we ingest bombard the body, overwhelming the internal system and

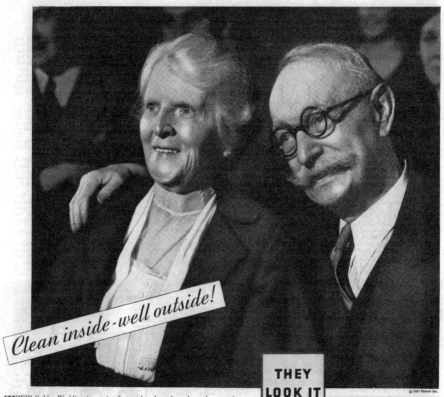

Clean inside-well outside!

THEIR Golden Wedding is coming fast, and here they are, having the time of their young lives, these two, as romance and love and adventure flash by them on the silver screen.

Health! Being glad to be alive, every day! Taking the years in their stride, with a smile!

This business of being *well*, which is the thing that makes life worth living, is not as difficult as most people make it. According to the doctors, the rules for most of us are few and simple: eat, exercise, and sleep right; keep yourself internally clean.

Doctors pretty well agree that (barring germ diseases) most illness and headache, most drowsiness, lack of pep and ambition, most cases of seeing the world through blue glasses generally, are due to failure to keep "clean inside." One famous British physician goes so far as to say "auto-intoxication (the self poisoning that comes when you are not internally clean) is perhaps the most important factor in the production of human disease."

Just as most doctors agree in blaming this condition for much of our sickness, so they also agree that the Nujol type of treatment is the safest way to relieve it. Crystal-clear Nujol can't possibly hurt you. It isn't a medicine at all. It has no drugs in it. It isn't absorbed—so it can't make you fat. It is colorless—tasteless—and children love it. And it costs so little!

The tonic effect of Nujol on your whole body is due to the way it helps you without using weakening drugs. Since it is harmless as pure water, many doctors advise taking it as regularly as you brush your teeth or wash your face. It's com-

mon sense, isn't it, that if you keep as clean inside as you do outside, you increase your chances of being well—and therefore happy—all the time? Remember two things if you want to enjoy "Nujol health."

One: Don't expect results overnight. This is nature's own method, and nature is never violent. Your body will respond gratefully, and day by day you will feel better as this soothing treatment takes effect.

Two: Be on your guard. Don't accept any substitute. Your druggist has Nujol—always in a sealed package—always trademarked "Nujol" so you will be sure to get it.

If you want to smile at the years, put yourself on the simple, natural Nujol treatment—and begin today!

Nujol

health

FIGURE 6. Advertisement for Nujol laxative. *McCall's Magazine,* 1931.

rendering it no longer able to purge itself of this onslaught. From this perspective, detoxification can act as a shield against the impacts of a polluted environment.

Similar to detox, and often described in similar ways or in tandem with purges, is "clean eating." Like the detox narrative, clean eating narratives revolve around a polluted environment, although in this case the pollution tends to be linked to fast-food diets. In his book *Clean Gut: The Breakthrough Plan for Eliminating the Root Cause of Disease and Revolutionizing Your Health,* celebrity health guru Alejandro Junger describes his conversion experience from a sickly "modern food" eater to a practitioner and proselytizer of a diet that includes a detox regimen that "rests" the colon, giving liver and kidneys the opportunity to clean out the toxins that creep into bodies through modern society's polluted environment and unhealthy lifestyles.

Many of these clean-eating stories begin with revelation narratives that parallel the stories of angels and bright lights of nineteenth-century awakenings. Junger's narrative follows the tenets of the conversion narrative closely, describing an "awakening" that includes a revelatory vision while visiting a Zen monastery.[9] Food reformers then present these encounters with new ways of life to others, didactically, in order to awaken their audience as well. Like Joseph Smith, Ellen G. White, or other nineteenth-century evangelicals, clean eating and detox advocates begin with a narrative of revelation, of awakening, that has led to a transformation in their ways of life. In other words, clean eaters repeat the romance of past reformers, perfecting the body through purification. A purified lifestyle becomes the way to save others and save the world. In a world where there are only two categories—inside-outside, nature-culture, discipline-pleasure—the romantic escape provides a way to reconcile contradictions: nature can save us from culture; local can save us from globalization; the artisanal can save us from the industrial; and detoxification can save us from a toxic world.

"[T]here are no high-quality clinical trials published in the medical literature supporting the use of regular or periodic colonic cleansing or purges to promote general health," concludes an overview of the scientific literature on these practices.[10] Detoxers, such as the *Food Matters* directors, Dr. Oz, and actress Gwyneth Paltrow vie with detox debunkers in the popular media, alternating titles like "21-Day Green Smoothie Boot Camp!" with "You Should Ditch the Desire to Detox." "[O]ur bodies have evolved to do a pretty damn fine job of getting rid of harmful stuff by themselves," states another popular online article. "There is no known way—certainly not through detox treatments—to make something that works perfectly well in a healthy body work better," stated detox-debunker Edzard Ernst in the *Guardian*.[11]

But whether or not yogurt, laxatives, colonics, purges, or other detox practices actually "work" is not the question here. Instead, the question is this: Why, despite a lack of evidence that these practices produce "health," has the idea of the "clean inside" repeated itself over more than a century of American life? In particular, why, as gastroenterologists have noted,[12] is this practice reemerging today, "discussed endlessly at dinner parties and discos," according to Bernard Dixon in *The Lancet?* "[T]his desire for purity," he states, is a "mass delusion that has spread from nowhere over the past decade and is now the subject of beliefs as firm as convictions that the sun will rise in the morning."[13] Whether or not detoxification should be "consigned to the dustbin of medical history," as Dixon advises, is less important here than the question of why a scientifically unproven health practice has reemerged, one that promises salvation through purification. If purity, like wilderness, is a mirror of our own "too much-ness," then detoxification becomes a symbolic boundary that protects us from this too much as a way to promote personal health: ill health is a product of contamination, and the solution is to heighten purification practices.

This bifurcated view of the world—with either its purified or its romantic side as the ideal—has become at best a waste of time and money and, at worst, physically and politically dangerous. Like the Northern European Yankee diet, which was presented as the ideal for much of American nutritional history, a diet that creates a symbolic boundary also creates a social one, in which the search for status puts the middle class on a treadmill of purification that can become debilitative. In the past, the treadmill of purity led to actual health problems in two ways: first, it ignored other healthy food ingredients in the diets of other people in other places. Many of those other diets contained, for example, greater amounts of fiber. The idealization of the Northern European diet resulted in a significant lack of fiber in the American diet, leading to actual health problems, and the need for those laxatives. Secondly, the treadmill of purity became tournaments of self-control, making thinness a sign of that control, with women particularly susceptible to the pressure to display their status through their increasingly purified ingestive practices, leading to eating diseases such as anorexia.[14] Finally, as the symbolic boundary between purity and danger led to the social boundary dividing "us" and "other," the more dirty bodily functions became associated with stigmatized groups of people, making "inner hygiene" even more important to status. Defecation and the fermentations of digestion became suspect and worth avoiding.[15] The health crazes of purging and colonic irrigation are the current practices based on this treadmill of purity.

Just as Americans turn to the treadmill of purity to heal themselves, they attempt to solve larger-scale issues with hyper-purification strategies. The Food Safety Modernization Act is an example of the treadmill of purity on a national scale.

SCALING UP DANGER: THE FOOD SAFETY MODERNIZATION ACT

In January 2011, President Obama signed the Food Safety Modernization Act (FSMA), one of the few bipartisan legislative successes of his administration. In the biggest overhaul of the food safety system since 1938, Congress responded to foodborne disease outbreaks by giving the Food and Drug Administration (FDA) powers to establish preventive procedures for monitoring "critical points" of agricultural production and food processing where microbial contamination was likely to occur. In part, it expands the sorts of monitoring and inspection mandated for livestock processing facilities a few years earlier. The legislation also gives the FDA greater authority to track the provenance of foods and to recall food declared unsafe.

The technology to follow the trail of contamination through DNA analysis has become very powerful. This became particularly clear when, later in the year that the FSMA was signed, several dozen people died from eating cantaloupe tainted with *Listeria*. New forms of scientific detection—and new funding for science labs to do the detecting—led the FDA to a Colorado farm that had recently dedicated an unusually large area, 480 acres, to growing cantaloupes.[16] Further review revealed that the farm had washed the resulting 1.5 million melons with a converted and unsanitary potato washer. Yet, the farm had received a "Superior" sanitary rating from a private inspector at the beginning of the harvest season.

The cantaloupe farm is just one of many places where deadly bacteria have been found in food and produce. Another well-known outbreak, in 2006, involved *E. coli* O57:H7 contamination of spinach that killed three and sickened at least two hundred in more than a dozen states. This outbreak led to a national recall of all bagged spinach. These crises were costly in terms of human health and in producer income—not just the producers responsible for the outbreak but every producer of bagged spinach, since consumers could not tell the difference between contaminated and uncontaminated produce.

These foodborne illness outbreaks led to a flurry of media coverage, consumer anxiety, and food safety regulation. As a result of the spinach outbreak, leafy green producers, in 2007, voluntarily designed a set of rules to prevent such crises in the future and many public universities and producer associations created "good agricultural practice" (GAP) programs that trained farmers to implement plans to control contamination. Supermarkets increasingly required their producers to implement these GAPs. Since these programs have been put into place, the number of outbreaks has dropped. "Food safety programs work, and there's definitive proof of that," states food safety scientist Keith Schneider.[17] The FSMA was designed to expand these successful food safety programs, setting standards and requiring farmers to carry out HACCP (Hazard Analysis and Critical Control Points) practices and plans that would maintain strong boundaries between clean and unclean food. The hope is that farmers, by keeping tight control over their production processes, can make clean food that will not kill or sicken consumers.

The problem is that only larger-scale farms can afford to implement these kinds of regulations. In response, Senators Jon Tester and Key Hagan submitted legislation that exempted smaller farms from the regulation. Yet, argues Schneider, "that doesn't matter because if they want to sell to the Walmarts of the world they are going to have to have a food safety program. There isn't a buyer on the planet who's going to allow anybody to sell produce without a food safety plan in place."[18] In discussions reminiscent of Progressive Era farm sanitation programs, small farmers have been targeted as the problem and consumer support for small farms as a threat to safety. For example, Steve Sexton argued on the *Freakonomics* blog that because large-scale industrial agricultural operations can afford to implement the kinds of HACCP practices mandated by the FSMA, they therefore are better able to protect consumers: "this kind of food contamination is less likely to occur at the large-scale farming operations that locavores love to hate."[19]

Yet, the cantaloupe case, looked at more closely, presents a more complicated picture. The Jensen brothers had vastly expanded their cantaloupe acreage to meet their newly minted contract with Walmart, their 480 acres representing nearly a quarter of the total cantaloupe production acres in Colorado that year.[20] It's not clear whether the Jensen brothers knew what they were getting into when they signed the Walmart contract, but they did change their packing shed processes to process more cantaloupe. It is likely they did this in order to accommodate the expansion in production acres. Did they promise Walmart more than they could actually deliver? Did the disease problem in this case come from farmers who were attempting to scale up to the industrial food chain? If so, then is it small farmers or the industrial food chain demands on farmers trying to scale up that caused the problem? While the Jensen brothers' farm wasn't small, they were new to selling cantaloupe on a large scale.

As the food system industrializes, retail supermarkets seek systems that are rationalized—that is, predictable, consistent, and sanitary. Supermarkets also want to work with larger operations, to lower transaction costs: lots of contracts and inspections with lots of smaller farms takes time. Yet, they also want to meet consumer demands for food from smaller, local farms. The tension between scale, safety, and efficiency means that supermarket chains buy from smaller local farmers but want them to get bigger.

Yet, agricultural production, particularly fruits and vegetables, doesn't fit into the industrial system. Rationalization of systems is how industrial systems grow into larger-scale enterprises. Creating these systems requires the setting of strong boundaries of control. However, fruit and vegetable-growing are processes dependent on nature, which is not necessarily predictable and consistent. Also, agricultural production is not the same as making widgets because it is embedded in the world and not behind a factory door.[21] Because agriculture is embedded in nature, it is not completely under human control. Scaling up production systems that are not completely controllable inevitably leads to conundrums: continual struggles to achieve the impossible. Nonetheless, supermarkets provide a pull for farms to rationalize the expansion of their operations in order to win profitable contracts. Supermarkets therefore provide incentives for farmers to scale up to larger enterprises that will meet industrial needs.

The Jensen brothers' farm has become the center of a debate about the role of small and large agriculture in food contamination. For some, like Steve Sexton, the Jensen brothers' farm was a small, locavore farm, and the problem was that consumers want small farm products and supermarkets are therefore forced to buy from these dangerous places. Some saw it as a large farm where the farmers made lots of mistakes. Others saw it as a problem of buying from cantaloupes not grown in the desert, where it doesn't rain and therefore where cantaloupes are less prone to contamination. Therefore, once again, supermarkets are pressured by consumers to offer local produce, which is

TABLE 1. Major Outbreaks of Foodborne Illness in Produce, 2011 and 2012.

Outbreak Source	Outbreak Details	Food Chain Relationship
Townsend Farms: "grow, harvest, process and deliver premium berries to stores around the country"	Pomegranate seeds from Turkey used in processed juice infected with hepatitis	Large-scale juice processor selling to supermarkets such as Harris Teeter
Izabal and Miracle Greenhouses, Mexico (large-scale greenhouses)	Cucumbers contaminated with *Salmonella*	Restaurants and other locations in several states
State Garden: "Producer of store brand private label salads, celery and cooking greens"	*E. coli* in spinach	Sells clamshell-packed spinach to several supermarket chains
Daniella Mangoes: one of the brands of Splendid Products, a large-scale shipper to supermarkets	*Salmonella*	Costco, Save Mart Supermarkets, Food 4 Less, Ralph's, Topco stores, El Super, Kroger, Giant-Eagle, Stop & Shop, Aldi, and Whole Foods
Chamberlain Farms: grew farm to 500 acres of cantaloupes	*Salmonella*	Large farm selling to Walmart and regional supermarket chains
Sprouts	*E. coli*	Sprouts in Jimmy Johns sandwiches—large food chain
Romaine lettuce	*E. coli* O57:H7	Farm selling to multistate supermarket chain for its salad bars
Turkish pine nuts	*Salmonella*	Sold in bulk bins at Wegmans grocery stores
Jensen Farms	*Listeria*	Farm accounted for nearly quarter of total cantaloupe acreage in state, sold to Walmart and Kroeger
Agromod papayas	*Salmonella*	Supplies to major supermarket and restaurant chains
Evergreen sprouts	*Salmonella*	Sold to major chains in several states
Del Monte cantaloupe	*Salmonella*	Sold to "national warehouse club"

SOURCE: Centers for Disease Control and Prevention.

more dangerous because it is not from California. That said, even California irrigated-desert farms have been linked to foodborne illnesses. The FSMA mandates the kind of rational control over nature that farms of any size and in any place can't always produce, even, sometimes, in the fairly sterile conditions of dry climates. This creates a sanitary treadmill, with supermarkets forcing consistency and scale-up that exacerbates sanitary problems, while the FDA, and the FSMA it is trying to implement, forces control over sanitation. The final product of this treadmill is a situation that encourages farms to grow larger so they can afford to implement the necessary safety systems.

Table 1 shows the major, multistate foodborne illness outbreaks traced to fresh produce in 2011 and 2012.[22] Of course, multistate impacts come from large-scale companies because their production goes beyond the local scale. Food safety experts argue that the smaller outbreaks, from the smaller farms, don't show up in CDC data. "Most of the smaller outbreaks on small farms you never hear about because only one or two of the people are getting sick."[23] Yet, that is part of the problem: Farmers' attempts to industrialize through large-scale production systems for fruits and vegetables that meet the needs of multistate supermarket contracts create intrinsic risks for consumers, who want both local and safe food. The needs of this food safety supply chain pressure farmers to industrialize further, in order to participate in these contracts. The nature of nature clashes with the needs of industrial food chains to produce food on a large scale that is completely free from disease. In fact, it promotes a system that will always create a potential scenario for large-scale foodborne illness. The expansion of industrial farm production creates these scenarios, and leads to conundrums about cleanliness. In other words, the conundrums around purity have led to regulatory solutions that will perpetrate the problem, leading to another treadmill of purity.

The Food Safety Modernization Act depends on setting strong boundaries between clean and unclean and strong controls over the natural systems that comprise agricultural production. But, even the experts assert that a pure and sanitary system is unattainable: "there are no particular amounts of these practices that produce 'safe food,'" states Jim Prevor on his *Perishable Pundit* blog. "We are talking about setting some level for each of these things ... this is at least as much a hunch as it is science, and the benefit derived is most uncertain."[24] Each foodborne outbreak has led to increased attempts to control the system, which only further increases the size of farms. This materialization of the treadmill of purity, in which farmers are asked to establish food safety regimes based on controlling that which is uncontrollable—nature—through sanitation, consistency, and predictability, attempts to rationalize operations in ways that are not possible because of agriculture's connection to nature.

Purification practices will lead to even larger-scale agricultural production systems. Experts agree that there is no way to make food completely safe. Yet, every outbreak leads to another round of purification requirements that don't necessarily purify but that do lead to the further shakeout of smaller farms. The ultimate end of this treadmill may be vegetables grown in vast "protected" production facilities—large dirt-free vertical greenhouses using hydroponics.

How can people rethink this relationship between purity and danger? One possible model is the National Organic Standards Board.

THE NATIONAL ORGANIC STANDARDS BOARD: CREATING IMPERFECT BOUNDARIES THROUGH DISCURSIVE GOVERNANCE PROCESSES

In 2002 a small Maine organic blueberry farmer, Arthur Harvey, sued the United States Department of Agriculture. He argued that the organic products offered to American consumers—like the cereal labeled "organic" containing nonorganic dried blueberries—weren't what they claimed to be.[25] Twelve years later, Alexis Baden-Meyer, the political director of the Organic Consumers Association, was handcuffed and dragged from a USDA organic food hearing as protesters chanted, "Don't change sunset!"

Both of these conflicts focused on a small, relatively unknown advisory body to the USDA's National Organic Program: the National Organic Standards Board (NOSB). A group made up of farmers, consumers, environmentalists, and members of the organic food industry, the NOSB's legislative mandate is to figure out where to draw the line between organic and conventional food systems. That is, the NOSB figures out what should be in and what should be out of the organic food production system by drawing a boundary between "synthetic" and "natural." This advisory board also determines what products are allowed in organic production because they do not have organic substitutes. These products are then put on a list, the National List of Allowed and Prohibited Substances, known in the industry as "the National List."

The Organic Foods Production Act, part of the 1990 Farm Bill, mandated the creation of national organic standards and the administration of these standards through the National Organic Program (NOP) housed at the USDA. The legislation specifically defined organic as agriculture "without the use of synthetic materials," with synthetics defined as "a substance that is formulated or manufactured by a chemical process or by a process that chemically changes a substance extracted from naturally occurring plant, animal or mineral sources."[26] The legislation also created the NOSB, a standing citizen advisory board composed of farmers, consumers, certifiers, scientists, industry representatives, environmentalists, and other stakeholders, charged with the job of advising the NOP on what should, and should not, be "allowable" in organic food. The NOSB's job, therefore, is to guard the boundary between organic and conventional food. Without that boundary, organic food ceases to exist, since the label "organic" loses integrity when any company can use the label without adhering to meaningful standards.[27] Once again, boundaries are important to the existence of the organic food system, but how to set those boundaries is a social question.

There are many different kinds of boundaries the NOSB must fashion. First, some materials don't have organic forms—baking powder for example. Second, there are materials that are not synthetic but are not yet produced organically, or in enough volume to meet the needs of organic producers. For those situations, the Organic Foods Production Act gave the NOSB the authority to recommend that substances be put on "the National List." These substances were allowed for a five-year period and then were "sunset," meaning they had to be reconsidered or dropped from the list.

To be able to use the words "USDA Organic" on a label, a food product has to contain 95 percent certified organic ingredients, and comprise less than 5 percent of the allowable National List ingredients in that food. When consumers hear about this list, they tend to feel a sense of betrayal. To consumers organic means organic, not a standard that is negotiated, not labels that aren't clear about the percentage of organic ingredients. Organic, to consumers, means pure. And when conflicts around NOSB boundary-work bring purity conundrums to light, the consumer loses faith in organic integrity: that what they are buying, at a higher price, is closer to what they value, and therefore worth more.

William Cronon tells us that the line between the natural and the synthetic is not discoverable "out there"—it is in fact a mirror of ourselves. Yet, organic food is legislatively defined as containing no "synthetic ingredients" (see the act's definition of "synthetics" above). Which means that the organic food industry has a conundrum: if in fact the boundary of purity is always negotiated, if these are bifurcations Americans have created for themselves, then the NOSB is a small group of people assigned an impossible project. Yet, this project is absolutely necessary if organic agriculture is to survive. Boundaries are impossible, but they need to be decided.

Separating organic from synthetic and nonorganic, and then allowing some of these substances into organic food, has been controversial ever since the establishment of the NOSB. On one side of the controversy are activists like Arthur Harvey, who believe that the rule should create a strong boundary between synthetic and "natural" ingredients. A libertarian pacifist who has not paid federal taxes since 1959, Harvey convinced the courts that the boundary between organic and conventional food had been breached. Yet, for Harvey, the boundary between synthetic and organic was only a proxy for his main concern: the corporate takeover of the organic food system. Harvey believed that, by allowing more and more synthetics into the National List, the corporations were creating loopholes that allowed what Michael Pollan has called the "organic-industrial complex" of large organic farms selling to supermarkets as the main purveyors of organic food.[28] As organic observers noted at the time, the larger food companies were buying up organic brands, and creating more processed organic food. As a result, the NOSB was faced with making decisions on more and more substances as these companies proposed more ingredients to be included on the National List.[29]

In the *Harvey v. Veneman* court case, the treatment of synthetic and non-organic substances, Harvey charged, was in violation of the Organic Foods Production Act. Harvey contended that the regulations provided a "blanket exemption" to processors, allowing them to use nonorganic substances in certified organic products if they were "not commercially available in organic form."[30] Lack of commercial availability, Harvey argued, was not a valid reason to allow individual organic processors to use a given nonorganic substance without NOSB review. The court agreed with Harvey on these counts and mandated new USDA guidelines and greater restrictions on the use of nonorganic and synthetic agricultural products. The court demanded that the USDA follow the OFPA-established procedure of submitting each synthetic and nonorganic ingredient to the National Organic Standards Board for review.

The organic economy's list of actors is diverse and their needs are varied and at times dissonant. For noncorporate actors in the organic economy, the survival of organic as a distinct alternative market represents more than a profitable brand. Organic producers seek to maintain their livelihoods, consumers seek to maintain their health, and organic social movement actors seek to maintain equality, environmental sustainability, and community resilience. The struggle to define organic shows that its survival as an alternative economy concerns more than just boundary setting to ensure purity. It is about maintaining the legitimacy of an alternative economy, the credibility of which depends on open deliberative civic processes in which these alternative food system actors go beyond simply creating a boundary between synthetic and organic, to the larger question of whether and how the market will meet their extra-economic needs.

On the other side of the controversy are the large-scale industrial producers themselves, who want a rule that is stable, enabling them to profitably invest in large-scale organic production processes to meet the mass market. This group finds the civic process burdensome and therefore wants to limit the amount of NOSB discourse and decision making. Since large food corporations have bought up most organic products that appear on supermarket shelves, these corporations now have a large voice in the NOSB process and tend to want more synthetics on the list. Not surprisingly, this group was also in favor of changing the NOSB sunset rules that led to the protest and the arrest at the NOSB hearing.

The Organic Trade Association (OTA) represents the interests of these larger organic processors. During the Harvey controversy, the OTA argued that stable standards would expand the organic market: "Market-led growth is only possible if organic farmers and processors compete on level ground with non-organic farmers and processors," OTA executive director Katherine DiMatteo stated. The standards, the OTA argued, should not be continually open to public debate. Instead they should "remain intact to minimize disruption and marketplace confusion and to protect the growing marketplace for organic farmers."[31] Large-scale processors could build profitable organic brands only if the NOSB created stable boundaries between pure and impure. By stabilizing organics, larger companies could make organic food into a tightly bound but highly-rationalized niche market, regulated by a fixed and stable set of standards, and designed to create an extra-profitable "brand."

The NOSB is therefore squeezed between actors who want a list of allowable substances that is regularly reviewed and large and powerful food corporations that lobby for a more stable and expanded list. In other words, the boundary is under continual contest, with some wanting the boundary to maintain strict purity and others wanting to make sure this niche market is profitable. In response to both groups, the NOP proposed a new set of more stable sunset rules for the NOSB, leading to written and active protests like the one that led to the arrest at the Texas public organic food hearing. The sunset changes, which include changes in majority voting and therefore would to some extent stabilize the list, open the USDA up to the charge that they are favoring larger organic producers and therefore helping along the growth of Pollan's "industrial-organic system." Yet, the NOP insists that the changes will make the process more transparent and more open to consumer concerns.[32]

Despite these forces pulling in seemingly opposing directions, and the current threat that new rules will undermine its deliberative and democratic nature, the NOSB is a promising example of an imperfect politics, a form of collaborative environmental governance.[33] Imperfectly, the NOSB seeks to resolve political tensions between actors by making decisions about boundaries between worlds, boundaries that in fact do not exist "out there" except through negotiation. The NOSB does so through a kind of "discursive governance," to create markets based on civic processes rather than the utilitarian laws of supply and demand. Organic markets need to be civic, that is discursively governed, in order to maintain their integrity. However, discursive governance is an imperfect form of politics that, in fact, intensifies the critique of the NOSB from both sides of the debate and threatens the legitimacy of organic in the mind of the consumer. Yet, the imperfect politics of discursive governance is the only kind of politics that will avoid the treadmill of purity. It is a costly, time-consuming, but necessary way to resolve political questions of sustainability in a world that increasingly needs to resolve those questions.

At the level of agency jurisdiction, the NOSB is mandated to represent the many actors in the organic food system: farmers, certifiers, processors, retailers, scientists, environmental advocates, and consumers, all of whom continually disagree with its decisions. Yet, it is through this continually contested process of discursive governance that the NOSB succeeds in maintaining the legitimacy of organic food. The only way for alternative economies to maintain their legitimacy is through ongoing civic discursive processes that negotiate organic modes of governance.

Some actors in this process recognize the importance of the NOSB's discursive role. For example, former NOSB chair Jim Riddle wrote an open letter to the secretary of agriculture in 2004, asking the NOP to restore "due process" in standards setting. Citing several examples, Riddle argued that the USDA had insufficiently incorporated NOSB and public input when deciding whether certain substances should be placed on the National List.

Riddle wrote, "I urge you to ensure that the NOP actually do what it is supposed to do under the OFPA and require that proper administrative procedures be followed when new policies, letters, and directives are formulated and new technical advisory panels are contracted."[34] During the legal contests around the *Harvey* case, organic food and agriculture groups, called "Friends of the Court," also supported NOSB's important role in maintaining a deliberative mode of governance. These same groups have also lobbied heavily against the new sunset rules.

Therefore, this little advisory board, which has little control over even the small segment of the food market for which it provides boundary advice, represents a much bigger issue: the potential governance of a possible future sustainable world. Under threat since its very inception, constantly under attack by both corporate and activist actors, and constantly making imperfect compromise decisions that please no one, this advisory group is unique among regulatory institutions in its ability to discursively construct an imperfect boundary between a conventional and an alternative production system. Despite these many weaknesses, the NOSB remains one of the most successful forms of discursive governance in the history of American alternative economies. Therefore, despite persistent threats against its continuation and capacities, the NOSB continues to hold hearings and examine technical data and public comments to recommend the addition or exclusion of particular nonorganic substances on the National List. Organic food system stakeholders large and small continually assail the NOSB for its decisions. Yet, it forces private actors into a public deliberative discussion of a food system that values something besides efficiency.

For example, at one point, organic processing companies went so far as to request the inclusion of over 600 nonorganic and synthetic ingredients on the National List. In order to quickly move through the National List review process for each of the 600 substances, and meet legislated deadlines, the USDA initially determined that a public comment period of a mere seven days would be sufficient. In this one week, the USDA received approximately 1,250 public comments, many expressing concern about the less-inclusive mode of governance demonstrated by the extremely short public comment period. In response, the USDA extended the public comment period to 60 days followed by an extended public hearing process that considered, and rejected, many of these substances.

Part of the strength of the NOSB—what makes it a discursive governance process—is its recognition that there was no way to determine the "true" bright line between synthetic and "natural" ingredients. At the March 2007 NOSB public hearings, National Organic Program personnel noted that they began their review of ingredients by trying to make a strong definitional distinction between synthetic and nonsynthetic ingredients, as well as between agricultural and nonagricultural ingredients. Yet, as NOP staff publicly stated, they abandoned their efforts to clearly define each of these categories. NOSB board members admit in public hearings that they are sometimes unsure about where to set boundaries. For example, at an NOSB hearing, one board member thought aloud: "When does an organic essence stop being agricultural, after how many cuts and splits? You know, where do we draw a line?" He asked industry to work with the board to determine "when does something stop being agricultural and become non-agricultural through the distillation process."[35]

Consequently the boundaries between synthetic versus nonsynthetic and agricultural versus nonagricultural remain somewhat ambiguous, and NOSB board members sometimes publicly disagree about how to classify certain ingredients. One contentious substance has been inulin / fructooligosaccharides (FOS). The inclusion of FOS on the National List represents an example of how the NOSB carries out its deliberative process of decision making and illustrates how deliberative public review is important to determining what is "inside" the organic food system. FOS are nonorganic / additive nutraceutical ingredients that, according to advocates, increase calcium absorption when consumed in yogurt. In her testimony in favor of including this substance on the National List, nutritionist Coni Francis of Stonyfield Farm argued that the NOSB should consider nutrition as part of its decision-making criteria. In her gloomy warning against its removal, she alluded to the prevalence of digestive diseases in America, as well as calcium deficiency among children: "Now, if we think that those of us who are in our 50s and 60s are looking at an issue with osteoporosis, I am very frightened about what's going to happen when these children reach their 30s and 40s."[36] She argued that reducing calcium deficiencies in the US population was a good criterion for including this substance on the National List.

Including nonorganic nutraceuticals on the National List according to Francis's health criteria did not go uncontested, however. Former NOSB chair Jim Riddle distinguished organic foods from "functional foods" such as nutraceuticals, arguing that "the side effects of a poor diet are not necessarily the responsibility of organic agriculture."[37] Functional foods and nutraceuticals often play a role similar to medicine in claims of preventing or correcting the effects of poor nutrition. Organic food producers, on the other hand, represent organic food as an inherently healthy alternative to nonorganic food rather than a corrective. This disagreement brings to light the contest between the agroecological and the nutraceutical definition of "good food." One promises consumer health and curative powers through ingredients while the other focuses on agroecological production systems.

In the end, the NOSB recommended adding FOS to the National List, based on claims of its functional health benefits. As the interim final rule states, "The inclusion of this non-digestible carbohydrate is thought to promote a more favorable intestinal microbial composition which may be beneficial to human health" (7 CFR Part 205). But using health claims as a basis to add a nonorganic ingredient to the National List clearly involves a significant rupture of boundaries to the criteria determining what is allowable in organic food and what is not. In this case, a "functional food" input definition of healthy food overrode the definition of organic food as free of synthetic ingredients. Other exempted ingredients, such as nonorganic fish oil, were also allowed because their ingestion increases omega-3 fatty acids in the product. In this case, the functionality of the food as an input has trumped the natural / synthetic boundary.

While this may seem like a defeat of organic philosophy, it also reflects how civic processes create foods based on different, and somewhat contradictory, interests and worldviews. Because the substances on the National List can be re-reviewed, the conflict between those who see good food in functional terms and those who see good food as coming from agroecological processes will, hopefully, continue to be a matter of public debate. For many critics of the NOP and the NOSB, judging organic food integrity in terms of ingredients rather than organic production processes already twists the playing field toward large corporations.[38] However, as Arthur Harvey indicated, to some extent the boundary between artificial and natural is a proxy for process.

Yet, the civic aspect of the NOSB discursive governance process can also fall into romance. The struggle over the role of pasture in organic milk production, which has been contentious ever since the establishment of the National Organic Program, is an example of how consumer input into the organic standards resulted in the creation of a romantic dairy system. The NOSB decisions on the Organic Pasture Rule are an example of how boundary making does not separate real objects and processes "out there" but in fact constructs the world through its boundaries. Consumers lobbied for an organic dairy system based on pasture "grass-fed milk," seen as reminiscent of earlier pastoral dairy production. Responding to consumer concerns, the NOSB created a new form of nature based on consumers' romantic notions of pastoral dairying as grass-based milk production. This purified pastoral is a romantic ideal of consumer nostalgia for an "invented tradition": a lost dairy system that never existed.

For years, the organic dairy industry was "working to secure clarification on organic milk production standards."[39] Noting that its action was "a result of comments, complaints and noncompliances," the USDA proposed a Livestock Access to Pasture Rule in October 2008 and finalized that rule in February 2010.[40] This rule mandates that cows producing certified organic milk must have a specific percentage of pasture-grazed grass as part of their diet. The two years of negotiations between the time of the proposed and final rule brought most actors into agreement as to minimum national pasture requirements of 30 percent dry matter and at least 120 days of pasture-feeding a year. But two parties, Straus Family Creamery and Aurora Dairy, took strong positions against the rule during the negotiation process.

The Straus-Aurora joint lobbying effort represents the ultimate example of strange organic political bedfellows. Albert Straus is one of the pioneers of organic dairying. Straus Family Creamery milks a few hundred cows and buys milk from a few other small local dairies, and was the first certified organic dairy company west of the Mississippi. Straus's local Bay Area following is intense, and a number of his consumers submitted comments to the USDA on the proposed rule, defending Straus's position.

Straus did not take issue with the fact that the ruling asks for a certain percentage of a cow's diet to come from pasturing *per se*. However, the Straus dairy is located in the Marin Agricultural Land Trust, and regulated by the California Regional Water Quality Control Board, whose water and land use quality requirements the farm must observe, particularly to maintain the water quality of the oyster beds in the ocean below the farm. Cows on pasture during the California coast's severe winter rainstorms can be tough on watersheds, due to agricultural runoff. Straus's operation exists in this fragile environment only because he works closely with local environmental officials on agricultural runoff issues.

Straus's political partner in this contest produces milk at the other end of the organic spectrum. Aurora Dairy, which operates mega-dairy farms in semi-arid Texas and Colorado environments, supplies the milk for many large supermarket private organic milk brands, such as Walmart, Safeway, and Costco. Grazing thousands of cows is clearly a headache, and in the past Aurora violated organic dairy rules to such an extent that even the Bush administration's lenient USDA was compelled to take action: in 2007 it sanctioned Aurora for violating the existing and loophole-ridden pasture requirements. Supermarket buyers seek to make their own-label organic milk brands more affordable by buying, once again, from larger-scale producers, Aurora in this case. Aurora is an ideal supplier for such products. To maintain low-cost operations, Aurora and other large-scale organic dairies have tended to shift the focus away from defining organic milk as grass-fed and toward a "pesticide-free" feeding standard. However, in so doing, these large-scale dairies have challenged the prevailing grass-fed consumer definition of organic milk.

Woes unite foes, and Straus and Aurora found themselves lobbying together, with Aurora clearly benefiting from Straus's greater organic reputation. The agroecological and industrial organic dairy operations found themselves on the same side of the fence as they argued the same point: pasture is complicated and costly and pasture rules should be more flexible. Yet they did so for different reasons and based on different agroecological organic dairy farming systems.

"A sustainable agro-ecosystem maintains the resource base upon which it depends," states agroecologist Steve Gliessmann, meaning that the operations of a sustainable agricultural production system must fit the context of its particular bioregion.[41] This is certainly true when it comes to pasture; the number of days of available green grass in any one place depends on soil, water, weather, elevation, and a number of other factors that vary from one region to the next. Yet the proposed organic rule set a national floor for the amount of pasturing that an organic cow must have, regardless of a region's agroecological circumstances. The USDA did respond to the Strauss / Aurora objections, by varying pasture requirements by region in the final ruling and allowing dairies to submit plans indicating how much pasture was possible in their particular environment. Yet, ironically, this flexibility, which Straus argued for in order to deal with local environmental issues, opened a door for more industrial, less agroecological dairies to compete with more agroecological dairy farms.

Once again, as with FOS, consumer demand shaped the meaning of organic milk in the contests over the design of this object. The USDA noted several times in the rule-making process that their definition of organic milk was the product of various consumer surveys, such as one by Whole Foods, showing that consumers identified organic dairy production with grass-fed cows.[42] Unlike most conventional commodities, consumers had power over how organic milk was produced and thereby influenced the design of organic production systems, even if, in the end, these systems do not always fulfill consumer imaginaries of what this production system should look like.

Yet, year-round fluid milk from pastured cows is an ecological anomaly, in which users (milk consumers) insist on a particular production system that fits their idea of traditional farm agroecologies and animal welfare. But this consumer interest in pasture-fed fluid milk draws on an imaginary production tradition. Pasture-fed dairying was traditionally seasonal, based on the ecology of grass that, in most regions, is available to cows only part of the year. Traditionally, pasture-based farms, that were known at the time as "summer dairies," produced milk seasonally, generally outside of city milksheds, for local cheese and butter factories. On the other hand, cows in the fluid milksheds serving cities produce milk all year long. They are bred and fed, in barns, for high production, eating the high protein necessary for this kind of high-production system.[43] Grass feeding of cows in fluid milksheds therefore takes one agroecology and tries to make it serve the needs of a different system.

Why do consumers have this power over the design of organic foods? Because consumers will only pay the organic premium price if they perceive organic products as legitimate. Romantic consumers imagine a production system that is entirely pure because the cows are out in nature. Organic integrity involves meeting the multiple visions of the actors—including romantic visions—in the alternative food system. These actors influence the system either through "voice," continuing to challenge the organic rules to live up to their production imaginaries, or "exit," no longer buying the product.[44] Producers, for their part, are thereby forced to design agroecologies not just to fit local environmental resources but also to meet the visions of other actors in the system, particularly consumers. The result is a struggle to fulfill consumers' romantic imaginaries of purity that dictate what organic farms should be like, in order to maintain organic milk prices. Correspondingly, if customers begin to feel that some organic companies are not meeting their production imaginaries, they become less willing to pay more for the organic product.

Consumers see grass-fed milk production as a return to nature when it is in fact a system that has never before existed in nature. In California's Central Valley, pasture requirements, ironically, encourage pasturing cows on irrigated alfalfa, often situated in areas with scarce water resources. To meet consumer fantasies about the nature of organic milk, producers end up scrambling to conform to consumer imaginaries rather than working to create agroecological food systems that are sustainable and make sense in terms of natural limits. Meanwhile, the large organic dairies, like Aurora and Horizon / Deans Foods, move in and out of court as organic advocates monitor their pasture-feeding practices and argue that these operations are barely keeping to the rule. Prosecutions in these lawsuits claim that large organic dairy operations are gaming the rules. Organic advocates argue that cows in these operations, milked 3–4 times a day, are mostly fed while milking and spend the mandatory pasture time outside simply digesting the high-protein feed they ate while being milked. According to one dairy farmer, "If a farm gets to the point of milking thousands of cows, 24 hours a day, the logistics of getting the herd from the milking facility to fresh grass, legitimately grazing—as required by law—becomes impossible."[45]

Consumers who want producers to fulfill their pastoral and personal health imaginaries should know that the notion of "consumer trust" in civic economies is agroecologically tricky. In civic markets, producers are sometimes forced to try to meet unrealistic consumer demands in terms of ecology, locality, animals, farmer-to-farmer, farmer-to-consumer, and farmer-to-government relationships. If consumers want the organic system to continue, they must understand the agroecologies behind organic production as reality and not as romantic pastoral imaginaries. If consumers really want to know "where their food comes from"—and if they want their milk produced through workable agroecological practices—they need to realize that agroecologies are contextual, and part of that context is political. Part of that is also natural—while we cannot separate society from nature, we also cannot separate nature from society. Yet, the fact that organic farmers and organic consumers sometimes have conflicting political interests is likely to make producers fear an open, civic discourse with consumers about organic-production agroecologies.

By the same token, if organic dairy farmers want to maintain their market, transparent and trustworthy communication with consumers about their local contexts will be necessary. Media accounts express consumer suspicion that "[t]he corporate takeover of organics, some say, is eroding the ethic that many take for granted as they throw an organic zucchini into the grocery cart."[46] Producers and consumers will need to be reflexive about their political interests and the degree to which they share production imaginaries. The organic food system as an alternative economy will only survive if consumers and producers participate in a public deliberative process that openly acknowledges these political and agroecological complexities.

The imperfection of civic markets means that the NOSB deliberation process is essential. If the boundary between organic and conventional agriculture is to be a matter of negotiation, the actors in this negotiation need to know the politics behind these decisions: the production imaginaries, changes in definitions of criteria such as "healthy," and the role of powerful actors like food corporations. The rules about transparency and inclusivity in creating organic boundaries are not perfect. And what gets talked about, and what does not—just working conditions for farmworkers, for example—is important. Yet, compared to other food systems, the civic nature of organic governance is a new kind of politics, a politics where the actors decide what is and what is not "inside" the organic food system. Participants in alternative food system civic processes have already decided to place boundaries around locality (such as Napa wines or French *terroir*), production processes (such as biodynamic), imaginaries (such as consumers' idea that cows should be on pasture), and fairness (such as fair trade products). These processes could be more open, discursive, and inclusive: for example, with regard to decisions about who gets to participate in a particular market, such as local farmers' markets, or who gets to sit at the table, such as farmworkers.[47] But as long as people try to change the food system by pursuing an ideal of purity, they will ignore discursive and civic governance processes as a way to move forward. Ideals of purity close down the discussion, create conundrums, and fail to lead to positive change.

Instead, we need to give up the idea that we are ingestive subjects, that a good life depends on maintaining boundaries of purity that make the false promise of safety. Instead, we need to be open to question and contest: we need to decide, together, when fences are necessary and where to put them up; we need to understand that these are socially constructed boundaries and we put these boundaries up aware that they create some problems while solving others. While these reflexive decision-making processes may not lead to perfect solutions, at least the stakes become clear, a part of the public conversation.

The treadmill of purity, on the other hand, is a threat to life and health. Romantic notions of pure food create unrealistic purification projects that, in some cases, lead to conundrums—continued attempts at creating boundaries that cannot be achieved. This creation of boundaries and purification of the inside leads to debilitation, both in terms of the internal ecologies of our bodies and the ecologies of the natural world in which we are situated.

Yet, boundaries and protection are also necessary—we want to avoid mixing food and fecal matter, for example, and some food safety regulations are necessary to do that. And the organic food system needs to be protected from the encroachment of the conventional food system, or else it loses its identity. How can Americans create new alternative food systems without falling into the treadmill of purity and without fetishizing safety and "the natural," while at the same time continuing to confront the problems with industrial food? This is a messy question, and the next chapters will show that, in order to answer it, people will have to do the messy work of rethinking the idea of free bodies and of what is within.

7

Ferment

AN ECOLOGY OF THE BODY

NOBEL PRIZE WINNER JOSHUA LEDERBERG has called the human body a "superorganism" of microbial communities.[1] Our human insides collaborate with millions of bacterial critters to make our bodies work. "[S]ome 90 percent of the protein-encoding cells in our body are microbes," states a *New York Times* overview of recent research.[2] Others have called our internal microbes the human "invisible organ." The bacteria in our bodies, combined, weigh as much as our liver. They don't just protect us, they are part of who we are; they are beings that evolved along with us, the same way we and our domestic animals evolved together.[3] In other words, there is no "us" without these microbial others. The other within us *is* us. Each human being is a biological community, a dynamic ecology. How do we better understand our relationship to our bacterial collaborators? How do we imagine our hybrid relationships with the animals inside us? To what extent are our innards a cultivated and productive garden or a wild and dangerous wood? And how do humans work through these questions to tell a different story about society and its politics?

The International Human Microbiome Consortium has begun to explore the superorganism of the human body. Through the consortium's Human Metagenome Project and the associated Human Gut Microbiome Initiative, researchers have embarked upon a lengthy project to discover the bacterial communities of which we are made.[4] As these bacteria become known, the consortium puts the computational capacities of systems biology to work to describe the human body, not as an autonomous, immune, and intact being but as an agroecological system in relation to the world around it. As a result, "the human body can be viewed as an ecosystem, and human health can be construed as a product of ecosystem services delivered in part by the microbiota."[5]

Even the skin, that symbol of protective boundaries, is being re-thought through new metagenomic discoveries. "The primary role of the skin," researchers admit, "is to serve as a physical barrier." However, they add, "The skin is also an interface with the outside environment and, as such, is colonized by a diverse collection of microorganisms—including bacteria, fungi and viruses—as well as mites." Therefore, "The perception of the skin as an ecosystem—composed of living biological and physical components occupying diverse habitats—can advance our understanding of the delicate balance between host and microorganism."[6]

But, in particular, researchers have discovered that it is our internal "enteric" bacteria that make our bodies dynamic, by moving what we ingest through our bodies. Researchers estimate that some 10^{13}–10^{14} microbes inhabit our gastrointestinal tract, representing more than a thousand species, and it is these alliances that help everything to "come out all right."[7] Biologist Julie Parsonnet calls the body a "human rain forest," and argues that humans are a microbial metabiome—a microbial community. In contrast to Levi-Strauss's description of cultures as defined by their diet, Parsonnet states, "We are what eats us."[8]

The boundary view of safety, with its focus on separating the pure from the impure, was supremely important to the rise of industrial society, whose increasingly urbanized citizens could not have survived without reforms like aseptic surgery and water purification. But new ideas of immunity acknowledge that living with microbes is as important as living without them. When our microbial ecologies are disrupted, the result is sickness, an increased tendency toward obesity, and a variety of other imbalances.[9] Without our bacterial alliances, the dynamic of our bodily system breaks down, creating blockages and crisis. Therefore, our eating is agroecological—what works depends on what is in us already, with different ecologies in different people. The comparative work has just begun, but initial discoveries indicate that different diets create different enteric ecosystems.[10] Enteric ecology is a new frontier.

PROBIOTICS: NEW BIOTA IN OLD BOTTLES

In spite of the connections being made linking diet and enteric ecosystems, the potential of this new relationship between the body and the world remains dormant. Instead, the current conversation about human bodies' relation to bacteria has continued to focus on separating out the good and the bad, with companies marketing the good bacteria to us as "probiotics": bacterial solutions to the usual problems. The marketing of Activia, a yogurt that purports to solve digestive problems, echoes that earlier era of laxative ads that claimed their product enabled the ability to "eat what you want." In one of Activia's ads, a soft guitar riff plays the company jingle with the logo on the screen, then switches to Jamie Lee Curtis sitting with her feet up on a couch the color of an Activia bottle. She holds up a newspaper. "First the bad news: 80 percent of this country suffers from occasional digestive issues like irregularity (she puts on an embarrassed face and rubs her stomach). No wonder. Our busy lives sometimes force us to eat the wrong things at the wrong times. Now the good news. I just discovered a yogurt called Activia that can help." Switch to a male voice and a picture of the Activia microbes forming into an arrow and moving down the picture of a woman's slim stomach, over which is printed "clinically proven with bifidus regularis." Lower down below her waist is the statement: "as part of a balanced diet and a healthy lifestyle." Then a male voice states: "Activia eaten every day is clinically proven to help regulate your digestive system in two weeks." Switch back to Jamie Lee Curtis: "The other good news? Activia tastes great." Smiling, she eats a spoonful of the yogurt. The screen switches to the product and the wording "Helps naturally regulate your digestive system" while women's voices in the background sing, "Activia!"

Jamie Lee Curtis is known for her sexy attractiveness. However, in the ad, her signature red hair is now gray. She therefore represents a market of older women who still want to look good (Curtis appeared topless on the cover of the American Association for Retired Persons magazine at about the same time that this ad aired). In some commercials, Curtis appears with various anonymous women who testify to the benefits of Activia, especially their experience after taking "the 14-day test" recommended in advertisements. The testifier admits to previous ignorance and to her awakening to the benefits of Activia—a form of commercial revelation. Curtis listens sympathetically and offers words of support.

The Activia commercials are part of a long line of testimonial advertisements dating back to nineteenth-century print ads. Like the early nineteenth-century patent medicine ads, probiotic merchants have adapted Romantic notions of salvation and the evangelical practice of personal testimony for commercial purposes. Dannon's claim that Activia will "naturally regulate" your digestion in a world so busy we "eat the wrong things" draws from the Romantic reform tradition of embracing nature to save us from a corrupt world. Finally, Curtis tells us we can eat what we want because Activia "tastes great." Activia is selling us American ideas of freedom: if we simply change our lifestyle practices we will be saved, and we do that by escaping our current degraded social world and embracing the outside, the microbe. This will give us more freedom—from busyness, from constipation—while giving us comfort as well.

The claims of probiotic companies remain controversial. In fact, in a lawsuit settlement, Dannon paid several million dollars as a fine for the overblown claims they made for their probiotic products. Nevertheless, the idea that probiotics can solve problems of constipation, immunity, and even, more recently, mood have become ubiquitous in the American media. Dannon's ads for another probiotic yogurt are aimed at children—or parents of children—and tell a story about friendly bacteria protecting the child from dangerous germs.

In one ad, three animated 3-D superhero characters play inside a refrigerator around bottles of Actimel. When the door opens, they run and jump inside the bottles. A boy grabs a bottle of Actimel from the refrigerator and drinks it. As he finishes the bottle, he makes yummy sounds and a protective halo surrounds his body. He says, approvingly, "Actimel!" Switch to pictures of the three superheroes who salute and respond in unison, "Team Actimel!" They are in various vehicles rushing their way to parts of his body. Switch to a scene where he is playing soccer. The ball is dirty and animated yellow germs jump from the ball into the boy, but the Actimel team fights off the ugly yellow germs as they try to attack the boy.

Activia ads claim to rescue digestion from the dangers of modern life by adding bacteria to the colon. In every ad, the narrator explains that Activia has bacteria that survive stomach acids and therefore colonize the body's nether regions. The "transit" of the bacteria to the colon is symbolized by a yellow arrow moving down a woman's body. Actimel (DanActive in the United States) contains what the company calls "L. Casei immunitas," a microbe that supposedly helps improve the immune system. In the Actimel ads, immunity is symbolized by a wall of good bacteria (little purple balls) bouncing away bad bacteria (big green balls). According to Activia and Actimel-DanActive ads, some microbes are on our side; they are friendly animals we can consume in order to free ourselves from constipation and contamination.

The Jamie Lee Curtis ad was so ubiquitous in 2008 that the weekly American comedy show *Saturday Night Live* did a very funny skit in which the Jamie Lee figure ate a bit too much of the yogurt and it had too good an effect. There are as many Activia spoof ads on YouTube as there are real Activia ads, many by young men, not the demographic featured in the official ads. Sarah Haskins makes fun of the representation of women in yogurt ads. "Yogurt is the official food of women," she quips, noting all the ways in which yogurt ads appeal to issues women can "generically relate to." Haskins's comedy video features conversations between two women who are enjoying yogurt so much that it reminds them of all sorts of other good stuff, like "private islands" and "not waiting in line for the women's room."[11] It is a food escape that parallels the men's hamburger ads catering to masculine identities. Most yogurt ads do speak to women, but the occasional ad tries to appeal to men as well, such as the Activia ad that features a fuzzy blue bear representing the "soft inner self" that men can take care of by eating yogurt.

In Activia, the serviceable microbe is called "Bifidus Regularis" and in Actimel it is "L. Casei immunitas." With these names, Dannon seems to have turned the Linnean classification system into a kind of branding mechanism. The real name of the Activia bacteria is the much less suggestive *Bifidobacterium lactis* DN-173-010. A global perusal of ads in the late 2000s shows Dannon and other companies promising that the good microbes in their products will alleviate the pains of irregularity, "overindulgence," aging, stress, weight, sluggishness, a feeling of unfemininity due to bloating, and a fulfillment of the needs of the "inner self," by eliminating the bad microbes that cause intestinal problems. These probiotics ads commercialize our insides with brands. The question is whether or not this private microbe is better than the common version in cultivating a healthy gut. Doctors have been particularly skeptical about Dannon's claim about its private bacterial strain: "I cannot effing believe people think Bifidus Regularis is a real name for a yogurt bacteria," one doctor blogged in reaction to this name.[12]

In fact, the claim that eating yogurt can change the ecology of one's colonic bacteria is controversial, and while it is becoming increasingly clear that the digestive system plays a significant role in immunity, it is unlikely that probiotic bacteria enable the eater to avoid aging or colds, or to resolve the problems of a life too busy to eat a good dinner. In fact, the lawsuits against Dannon have challenged the company's claims about the benefits of this yogurt and in doing so have forced Curtis's ad off the market.

In contrast to this vision of private bacterial strains doing extraordinary things, wildlife ecologists have discovered that it is not that easy to introduce a new being into an ecological system. That being needs to find enough to eat and live, which means that the being must find enough to eat in that environment. So, unless the microbes find an unused niche of edibles or manage to outcompete a species occupying a certain niche, they will simply not be able to live in that system.

These stories about our partnership with our own internal bacteria against a dangerous outside world also have a military flavor to them. Anthropologist Emily Martin has described how scientists talk about HIV as a martial story of good blood cells fighting bad viruses.[13] In the gut, the martial story is similar: lactic acid bacteria—supposedly the "good" colon bacteria—produce peroxide which, acting as homeland security, kills off other kinds of "germs," eliminating the terrorists in our own bodies.

Yet, the metabiome discoveries tell us that our bodies are not a garrisoned system but a collaboration with other beings, inside and out. We can try to manage our internal ecologies like a zoo, introducing species, like probiotics, to meet our needs. However, our internal nature is much like external nature: it resists our attempts to make it completely subservient to our needs. Our internal selves include beings that have selves of their own. To see the body in this way can help us rethink our reliance on ingestion as a definition of virtuous citizenship. Digestive fermentation will always be dangerous because it troubles, with its messy dynamism, the ingestive imaginary of freedom as choice and control. No wonder the virtuous classes even rejected, at one point, the fermentation of yeast in bread as dangerous and worrisome.[14]

Our internal microbes are in a sense companion species: like dogs, they have evolved with us and have a symbiotic relationship with us while still being very much themselves. Extending the comparison, microbes can be like lapdogs, working dogs, or watchdogs.[15] They can also be the wild dogs that run in packs and chase you down, the ones you need fences—or gloves and soap—to protect you against. But the probiotic ads do not tell this more complex story of our relationship to our internal companion animals. Instead, they build on the idea that probiotic yogurt is just another ingestive product to help purify and protect us, to build immunity against the bad things, against stress, hard work, bad food, our own slovenly eating habits, and so on.

The obsession with ingestion—with "we are what we eat"—has been limiting the imaginaries of social change, making it difficult to deal with today's problems. Social reformers who try to change the world through ingestive imaginaries focus on the enforcement of boundaries between inner purity and outer contagion, fixing social change imaginaries into the static, binding forms of purification or romance. Both of these static imaginaries require political exclusion and lead to inequalities of status and distinction. Eating the natural, or the pure, will not save the world. Neither will an orthocratic politics that depends on imaginaries of purity and danger as a metaphor for social order.

AN AGROECOLOGY OF THE BODY

These attempts to control our intestinal species sound a lot like the now-discredited wildlife conservation policies decried by ecologist Aldo Leopold nearly a century ago. In *A Sand County Almanac,* Leopold explored the parallels between the purification of ecosystems through the elimination of animals like wolves and the sanitation of modern life through purification and boundaries. Leopold's chapter of the *Almanac* entitled "Thinking Like a Mountain" describes the attitude of forest managers in the 1940s: a good wolf was a dead wolf, a good environment was one purified of predators that feed on "good" species like deer. Leopold illustrates the consequences of an ecological management approach based on eliminating wolves:

> I have watched the face of many a newly wolfless mountain, and seen the south-facing slopes wrinkle with a maze of new deer trails. I have seen every edible bush and seedling browsed, first to anaemic desuetude, and then to death. I have seen every edible tree defoliated to the height of a saddlehorn. Such a mountain looks as if someone had given God a new pruning shears, and forbidden Him all other exercise. In the end the starved bones of the hoped-for deer herd, dead of its own too-much, bleach with the bones of the dead sage, or molder under the high-lined junipers.[16]

At the end of the essay, Leopold goes a step further, to make a larger point about how this "too-much" infiltrates politics, because environmental management is also a mirror of a larger politics:

> We all strive for safety, prosperity, comfort, long life, and dullness. The deer strives with his supple legs, the cowman with trap and poison, the statesman with pen, the most of us with machines, votes, and dollars, but it all comes to the same thing: peace in our time. A measure of success in this is all well enough, and perhaps is a requisite to objective thinking, but too much safety seems to yield only danger in the long run. Perhaps this is behind Thoreau's

dictum: In wildness is the salvation of the world. Perhaps this is the hidden meaning in the howl of the wolf, long known among mountains, but seldom perceived among men.[17]

Here, Leopold extends his argument beyond wolves and deer, taking a cue from the barren mountain as to what can happen when people seek to avoid danger in the wider society.

Like Churchill's "Sinews of Peace," Leopold's essay took shape at the end of WWII, yet with a very different perspective.[18] Leopold quotes Thoreau, correctly using "wildness" and not "wilderness," and what he means in using this quote is not the romantic preservation of wilderness but a call for a world not built solely on safety and comfort. In the long run, he argues, trying to rid the world of danger—a politics of purification through elimination—simply brings more danger, more barren mountains and crisis-ridden societies. Like our ideas of ecological management through elimination, the broader politics of elimination—about getting rid of bad people, bad institutions, bad practices—is a mirror, an imaginary of self, a way of telling stories about ourselves. Leopold attempts to tell a different story.

What would Leopold's "wildness" approach to an embedded bodily ecology look like? How could dietary advice work toward a balanced enteric environment that would solve social problems in more environmentally complex ways? It would require that we think about bodies differently, tell different stories about how we deal with our choices. Ingestion is a simple story about purity and danger; digestion is a more complex story about how we relate to the world.

If we look carefully at the recent discoveries of the human metabiome, we may gain new ways of thinking about our internal ecologies. Despite ferment's ancient origin, research in this area is young. In particular, the fermentive microbial relationships of the earth's soil are still a vast unknown: "The evidence for soil biodiversity as an asset for farmers 'working with nature' to achieve sustainable production in a way which is valued by society at large, is still scant."[19] Similarly, our internal ecologies are still a mystery: "Studies that attempt to associate complex diets with changes in the microflora and disease are virtually nonexistent."[20] In fact, the intestinal metabiome has been called "a new frontier in molecular biology."[21] While we know so little about the microbiotic world in which we are imbedded, the idea that the human self is a living collaboration points politics in new directions. Rather than thinking of the world as composed of purities and dangers, and of a good world as one with a strong boundary separating the two, the metabiomic body teaches us to think of the world as composed of "socio-natural objects," created through the relationship between humans and nature.[22]

The new microbiome research gives us a way to rethink ourselves as citizens. One of the body's most important socio-natural objects is shit. Primarily composed of bacteria, this collaborative by-product is what comes out of an alliance between our food system and our internal ecologies. Seeing shit in this way enables us to see how our lives are fermentive processes that create socio-natural relationships.[23]

We can become "digestive" rather than "ingestive" subjects, part of a network of influences that is more complex than simply separating the world into "for us" or "against us." In the words of science studies scholar Michel Callon, we and microbes are part of a "hybrid collective,"[24] in which human-animal relationships are more complicated and more dynamic, in which we transform ourselves and each other through these relationships.[25] In other words, by rethinking our relationship to our own bodily political ecologies perhaps we can also rethink our relationship with each other. Adopting the imperfect politics of ferment would require us to go beyond defining health in terms of boundaries and safety and, instead, to make imperfect alliances with not always trustworthy or competent actors and institutions, such as bureaucrats, businesses, nonprofits, and other people of questionable motivation who seek public consent. A world where people cling to safety will not be fully safe, although someone will always be willing to offer us such a safe world if we will simply fork over something precious in return, often money or obedience. False dichotomies make for false promises. Will government, "third parties," or "networks" truly guarantee safety? No narrative is completely true, and believing too fully in any one of them leads to hopelessness. Only by embracing a messy, imperfect social change politics is it possible to avoid the messianic promises of purity and romance.

Contemporary fermentive political ecologies do not come from protective boundaries or martial alliances but from collaboration with those who have different ideas about a good world. Those collaborations involve internal transformations that require letting go of the idea of an intact self protected from the outside. A political ecology of ferment allows for multiple narratives about the world, based on very different definitions of a good way of life.

The digestive imaginaries of complexity that we need in order to understand our own bodies parallel the kinds of complex social imaginaries necessary for understanding the complex paths to be taken to reach alternative futures, and the human role in choosing those futures. Only by understanding that current society is complex, contradictory, dialectical, and full of trade-offs will it be possible to make a better future. Fermentation, as a new metaphor for the complex, messy politics of today, may, therefore, help provide new narratives of social change.

In these new narratives, food advice and politics are, as usual, parallel: Americans can create their own good food through inclusion, through microbial stews in their own political kitchens, rather than embracing an imagined outside of Tuscan peasant food or Bifidus Regularis. American ideas about a healthy society should include attention to what is healthy about the historically stigmatized American cuisines, about beans and greens, about cornbread as opposed to corn syrup, about the way the lime in tortillas releases good amino acids when combined with corn, and all the mustards and the turnip greens which, it turns out, provide pasture for internal biodiversity. This politics respects Europe and its food traditions but pays attention to the idea that the sacralization of European diets excludes other equally healthy diets—and the people who eat them—that are part of American dietary history but which have been, until now, deemed inferior or rendered invisible.

Fermentive political ecology enables democratic citizens to tell a different story about how to create a more healthy society. A fermentive approach embeds in the human body the fact that social change is intrinsically tied to a politics of social justice. For example, today's food reformers need to understand that their efforts to "raise the awareness" of others about healthy eating implies an unequal relationship in which some have intrinsically raised themselves above the rest.

The new biological understandings of the human body can help new, more fermentive social movements meet this challenge. Yet, very few social thinkers have considered digestive processes as a part of social life. Once we have eaten food, Arjun Appadurai's "subtle cosmological propositions" and the "collective representation[s]" of food seem to disappear. Food, once eaten, seems to be asocial. Yet, the fermenting that occurs in digestion is completely social, a collaboration between humans and the microbes they have domesticated, and which have domesticated them. It is about how people can live as a part of the multitude of beings, with a body that is a collaboration with these beings. This viewpoint avoids dualistic orderings and instead understands social change, and bodies, as a process rather than a category, a purity, or an ideal. If ingestion provides the metaphor for the authoritative nutritional narrative about safe and pure choices, and the dangers excluded, digestion is the imaginary that shows how to live in a world that cannot be categorized into "good" and "bad." Instead, it provides a different kind of subjectivity—a different way of being and acting—as part of, rather than protected from, the world around us.

In other words, a digestive subjectivity enables those interested in social transformation to get beyond problematic purity discourses, to understand human alliances with the less than pure world in which we live, the ambiguous choices we face, and the uncertainty of the civic processes necessary to make good decisions together. Digestion allows for the risky but productive mixings of ferment, as opposed to the purist ideas of homogeneity, uniformity, and sanitation.

This different kind of subjectivity leads us beyond thinking about society as an intact body with a mouth. Feminists have suggested that the body has "voice."[26] The "voice" that emerges from a digestive subjectivity is, like the science of the metabiome, a mysterious world we know so little about. But it points to a new way of thinking about society that is not built on inclusion and exclusion but instead on openness and collaboration.

We are always making Faustian bargains with our food, although the microscopic beings like *E. coli* H7:o57 sometimes change the conversation. Stasis and connection are conversations that are global, national, local, and internal. Digestive subjectivity may point to new ways of thinking about war, terrorism, or other threats to safety and security. It could help provide new narratives of social change dynamics that emphasize connection and transformation. It could help support new ways of creating a better world beyond the usual reform project of bifurcation and purification. It could get those interested in social change off the treadmill of purity. It could help create social movements that do not depend on defining an ideal and then attempting to convert others to this ideal, to bring them "inside." Instead, it allows for a narrative of social change in which different people with different ideals can come together and act with mutual respect. Digestive subjectivity points to a different way of looking at politics, as civic action that goes beyond the creation of an ideal, purified, protected society. Instead, it shows us how we can muddle through to a better but never perfect world, a fermentive, imperfect politics.

The digestive story is also about living with the choices already made: How to deal with an industrial economy that destroys our climate, wars that have no clear endpoint, and ways of life that do harm? Is there a kind of protection that does not create stasis and impose violence on others? Digestive subjectivity may make evident better answers to those questions.

This other kind of politics has, in fact, always been present in American society. Gary Gerstle, writing about the history of racial politics in the United States, describes two major political traditions in the United States: civic nationalism and racial nationalism. Civic nationalism, although flawed, has tended toward more inclusionist definitions of democracy. Reform movements based in this tradition have tended to distribute the benefits of American society more broadly, with a tendency—not always fulfilled—to see all humans as deserving. Gerstle argues that the civil rights movement and the integration of the military are two examples of this type of civic nationalism. The politics of racial nationalism, on the other hand, has tended to narrow the definition of who is deserving and to monopolize resources for that group. One of Gerstle's examples of racial nationalism was the monopolization by whites of New Deal agriculture program benefits. More recently, as the overt racism of purity has become less acceptable, racial nationalists have used ideas of threat and protection to justify control of others not like themselves, and to claim that these others are undeserving of the benefits of American society.[27] On the other hand, the politics of ferment is inclusive—allowing a broad and egalitarian ability to question our current society. Fermentive politics creates a more civic conversation about "the good life" through an ongoing, inclusive, and therefore contested and imperfect, egalitarian, democratic politics of "discursive will formation"[28] of the "deliberative turn"[29] or "reflexivity."[30]

Many of today's questions about social justice deal with boundary making and revolve around issues of citizenship and belonging.[31] Fermentation does not deny the importance of these boundaries; it is not another term for the "melting pot," that metaphor for assimilation. "We must find some other way of securing legitimacy," social justice philosopher Will Kymlicka states, "one that does not continue to define excluded groups in terms of an identity that others created for them."[32] Instead, fermentation is what happens when autonomous groups define themselves but also come together to make a third thing, in the same way that bacteria come together to make bread, beer, or the human body. It is a materialist parallel to the social justice politics of collaboration, of working with those unlike oneself to create something new. Fermentation can also create new kinds of safety, not based on sanitation and purity. Fermentation is, after all, what has traditionally kept milk products like cheese "safe" to consume before sanitation and refrigeration. Fermentation is risky and, like collaborative political processes, is always somewhat uncontrolled and unpredictable. It is, however, tolerant of mistakes. It also involves trust, because of its unpredictability and imperfection. A fermentive politics is open to social justice perspectives around "tolerance,"[33] "recognition,"[34] and "respect."[35] It enables people to maintain their group solidarities while working with others who don't share those commitments.

Digestive subjectivity does not reject an emancipatory vision of social justice. Unlike those who argue that "freedom" does not exist, digestive subjectivity points to freedom as process, not ideal: definitions of "the good life," particularly in this case "good food," reflect both civil society notions of democratic representation and broader notions of equality in terms of membership, especially inclusive membership of those most stigmatized by purity politics.

Whether it is peace in the world or sodas in schools, a politics that starts with defining "good behavior" and then transforms the world through "behavioral change" is a politics of "conversion."[36] It is apolitical in that it cuts off any negotiations about what good behavior is, since the goal—the perfection— has already been defined. It is also a politics of inequality since "good" behavior tends to be located in the practices of the elite who define themselves as the deserving. As the previous chapters have shown, dietary advice mirrors this politics. Rethinking people's everyday relationship to food can create different habits of life, ones that encourage reflexivity, plural knowledges, and a recognition of the social and material complexity of our current problems.

A digestive imaginary gives those interested in changing the world a way to think outside of dualistic orderings and toward the world as dynamic processes. If ingestion provides the metaphor for a narrative about safety, the dangers excluded, digestion stories tell us about how people live with the choices they have made. Digestion is the story of the world made through alliances and the uncertainty of that process. How will this partnership manifest itself? Will it be pleasant or painful? Will the choices made enrich or destroy? Will our choices lead to cheeses, wines, and other ferments, or will they lead to deadly *E. coli* that sneak into spinach, or the bird flus scientists warn will inevitably plague humanity? Will humans manage this globalization project they have embarked upon, this world of risky mixings between people and between people and things?

The social world, in other words, is already a product of risky mixings, of unpredictable complexities. Yet, without the embodied vision to imagine these mixings, people cannot respond, leading to crises they cannot resolve and an inability to move forward. The metaphors of process, of realist politics, of uncertain consequences, of dealing with the rich but challenging social and interspecies brew of humanity, are a productive contamination. Digestion is about the mess humans have gotten themselves into and how they can work through this mess as partners in a dynamic of transformation.

Climate change is one of the most insistent of these messes. Yet, we have no ways to think about transformation beyond the romantic embrace of alternatives and new styles of life. These romantic reform policies are often badly imagined and based on simplistic metaphors of social life that seek to reject, to eliminate the old objects and bring in the new, romantic Alternative. More complex, digestive metaphors of change could go beyond romance to bring to light other social options that may enable humans to live through and survive current environmental predicaments.

The politics of ferment is no doubt dangerous, and digestive subjectivity is on dangerous ground, but this way of thinking about the world can be liberating in ways that go beyond the modern ideas of freedom. Importantly, our fermentive collaborations push toward the egalitarian because, unlike sanitation politics, digestive politics has no one moral ideal, no one group that meets this ideal in charge of creating categories, no one trying to control others to meet this ideal, and no status distinctions that separate people into superior and inferior social statuses based on social ideas about purity. As the historical chapters have shown, sanitation provided the metaphor that justified these inequalities, while a politics of fermentative, digestive subjectivity creates more egalitarian ways to relate to each other and to nature, focusing on the complexity and hybridity of the socio-natural world.

The creation of a fermentive food politics will require that food reformers become less didactic and more civic, that is, spend less time convincing others of "good food" and "the good life" and listening more to others' ideas of good ways to eat and live, staying open to deliberative, public processes that take into account all of the interests involved in making a decision as to what is important and what is not. In this way, boundary setting is open to question and contest. While these contests may not lead to perfect solutions, the nature of the struggles and contradictions behind each mode of governance becomes clear, a part of the public conversation. The question becomes: How can politics move from sanitation to fermentation? A first step is the subject of the concluding chapter.

8

Toward a Fermentive Politics

STUDENTS IN MY GREEN GOVERNANCE class are looking through a choice of packages. I have asked them—in this first-day-of-class activity—to rank the packages according to their definition of "sustainability." Each begins by doing an individual ranking. I then ask them to boil down these decisions into a set of criteria he or she used in the ranking. Next, I ask them to rank the packages again, this time as a group. They tend to find, in the group, that different students rank packages differently and according to different criteria. Yet, I have asked them to make decisions together, to somehow come up with a joint ranking.

In the years of assigning this activity in my Green Governance class, I have found that students fulfill it in different ways. Some students focus on the package-rankings they have in common and rank those highest, while ignoring the disagreements. Others look at and discuss the criteria they used, and then decide on joint criteria to rank the packages. Sometimes, a student will make a powerful argument in favor of a criterion the others hadn't considered—for example, to include a social justice criterion that takes into account whether the worker was likely to have been paid adequate wages to make the package. Students reflect on these arguments and sometimes adopt this new criterion as their own. Other times, students aren't convinced by others' arguments and stick to their own criteria, agreeing to disagree. Sometimes, one of the more technical students—using scientific information to make a technical argument—explains how a certain package is not really as sustainable as it might at first seem, and the students may then jointly decide whether the technical information is important and whether they should move the package lower in the rankings. Sometimes they don't. Sometimes students simply vote on the ranking, without considering the criteria behind it.

At the end of the exercise, the students expect me to tell them the "right" ranking and the best process by which to jointly rank the packages. My job is to show them why there is no right ranking and that each process they used was a way to make joint decisions when they couldn't agree on a single definition of sustainability. This class exercise is meant to show students that there is no "pure" sustainable ideal, and that there are many different processes to get to a more sustainable world.

SUSTAINABILITY AS A WICKED PROBLEM

The lack of any one "right" definition of sustainability, or any one right process by which humans are going to make the world more sustainable, means that sustainability is a "wicked problem." It is a problem unsolvable by the orthocratic politics of purification or romance. Human existence now exceeds the carrying capacity of the planet. Technology and science have made this possible through processes of purification and sanitation that have improved many lives but now threaten our future as a species. This paradox is the foundational wicked problem of this era, what some are calling "the Anthropocene." Those who focus on how we will survive the inevitable loss of nature argue that the kinds of scientific knowledge and purification processes that got us into this mess are not the way to get us out. We need new ways of making knowledge, together.

The kinds of jointly made knowledge necessary to create a more sustainable world will require different knowledge-making processes. "A wicked problem," Valerie Brown et al. state, "has to be approached as an open system, one in which there are multiple views of how the world works and diverse ways of constructing new knowledge."[1] Sustainability scholars Silvio Funtowicz and Jerome Ravetz call this kind of knowing process "post-normal science." They compare this kind of process to conventional science, which involves "the study of an isolated piece of nature that is kept unnaturally pure, stable and reproducible." In contrast, "post-normal science" is the kind of knowledge-making process that is necessary "when uncertainties are either of the epistemological or the ethical kind, or when decision stakes reflect conflicting purposes among stakeholders."[2] They acknowledge that "our technology and medicine together have made nature predictable and in part controllable, and they have thereby enabled many people to enjoy a safer, more comfortable and pleasant life than was ever before imagined in our history. The obverse side of this achievement is that it may well be unsustainable, not merely in terms of equity, but even in terms of sheer survival."[3]

Creating knowledge for public decision making under our current conditions—high stakes, high uncertainty, high disagreement on foundational principles—requires post-normal science. The packaging lab activity discussed at the beginning of this chapter is meant to represent this kind of problem and to train students in this kind of decision making. In this post-normal process, "the traditional fact / value distinction has not merely been inverted, in post-normal science the two categories cannot be realistically separated."[4] To open science to these other forms of knowledge making requires the inclusion of "extended peer communities," including laypeople and other nonexperts. Bruno Latour describes this kind of scientific knowledge-making process as a "collective experiment" in which, for example, medical patients "now routinely generate their own science policy."[5] In medical arenas like HIV research and in environmental and food policy issues, this kind of "popular epidemiology"—the different, local, situated knowledge created by public nonprofessionals—has taken its place in public decision-making processes. In the same way, my students sometimes pay attention to the technical facts when making decisions in the packaging lab, and sometimes make decisions based on other considerations.

THE WICKEDNESS OF SUSTAINABLE KNOWLEDGE: ORGANIC STRAWBERRIES

How do we go about making this kind of knowledge: the wicked, undefinable, multi-situated knowing of sustainability? The difficulties are substantial. Consider the strawberry farmers who met over the course of two years to put together a manual on organic strawberry production. University of California agricultural researchers and cooperative extension agents came together with strawberry growers to put their knowledge into a document that could be disseminated to others. The institutional mission of cooperative extension is to increase agricultural production and farm income. Organic strawberries are a high-value crop and some consumers—especially parents with children—are paying extra for these strawberries because environmental groups tell them that conventional strawberries have dangerous pesticide residue. Other consumers concerned about the environment are willing to pay extra to reduce the hole in the ozone layer caused in part by the soil fungicide that has been used in conventional strawberry production: methyl bromide. Some consumers are willing to pay extra because they are concerned about farmworker safety, preferring strawberries produced without worker pesticide exposure.

Yet, when the strawberry group begins to talk about one kind of organic practice—the use of "trap crops," a technique that involves planting other crops near the fruit to tempt the pests away—the conversation becomes complicated. The extension agent does not see enough scientific testing of this technique to prove that it works: "We need to get that knowledge systematized," he states. A grower, on the other hand, responds that his commitment to this technique is not based on scientific reports. Instead, he depends on what he calls "outside info": "what farmers do around their pickups. I put a lot more store in what a farmer says than what a researcher says. If you have the two, what I do is ask farmers whether the research works in the field." The extension researcher, wanting to incorporate into the manual the kinds of knowledge the farmers respect, tries to bring the "outside knowledge" inside: "organic growers are carrying a big burden of observational knowledge. Local knowledge and local heterogeneity makes all the difference." The participants in the conversation devise a way to do this, which they call the "Farmer John" box: a separate text in the book for the kind of knowledge farmers bring to organic strawberry growing that has not yet been fully demonstrated in scientific research: "There are some ways in which we can keep the creativity of this," the extension agent states. But another participant, a research scientist, is worried about committing to a technique that is not scientifically proven: "The credibility, we have to deal with that."[6]

The participants in this conversation were dealing with "tacit" knowledge— local ecological knowledge, and farmer-around-pickup knowledge that is hard to stabilize in the more codifiable technical facts gained through systematic research practices. The conversation shows that farmers and researchers have different ways of judging the legitimacy of the knowledge they use, to some extent because local knowledge is specific to a particular production ecology and not universalizable to all the readers of the strawberry manual, and to some extent because the techniques and strategies have not been put through the scientific legitimation process of testing and peer review. For the researcher, the knowledge is not yet systematized, and more research—and more resources devoted to this research—will create the necessary knowledge to go into the manual. But the farmers don't see it that way—no matter how much scientist testing and peer review happens at the university or in the experiment station, they will not trust that knowledge until their *own* peers—other grower-farmers—say that it works in the field.

The farmers' lack of trust in the knowledge disseminated by agricultural scientists and university extension agents is not new.[7] However, conventional agricultural research, the "package" of seeds, fertilizers, and pesticides developed by scientists, public and private, is more "codifiable"—that is, it can be communicated through a manual—and is less sensitive to local conditions, ecologies, and histories. Disseminating the knowledge of conventional agriculture is simpler, since it is more universally transferable across ecologies, based on scientific research that can easily be communicated through a manual. Agroecological techniques, on the other hand, tend to rely on keeping pests and their predators in balance in a particular farm field with a particular local ecology.[8]

Organic farmers in the strawberry manual conversations made fun of their former days of "spray and pray," but they sometimes also waxed nostalgic for the conventional system that seemed to promise more guarantees and therefore less risk. These very sophisticated and expert grower-farmers know that the guarantees of conventional agriculture are also not necessarily reliable, at least not in the long run, but that didn't prevent them from wishing that their enterprises were more predictable, less risky. "We may 'know' how to grow organic strawberries, but we will never be able to know it in ways that match all the capabilities of the conventional system, in terms of its guarantees," the extension agent admitted.[9]

Because sustainability is a wicked problem, sustainable agriculture, renewable energy, smart cities, and new modes of mobility need to be "civic": ways of living that are dynamic, defined through inclusive public participation and ongoing, reflexive ways of making new knowledge that is open to social discussion and interpretation. These interpretations vary according to each actor's "situatedness": their position in the world, their family, occupation, training, community group, ethnicity, history. The Green Governance class lab activity is a hands-on learning process that teaches students both that sustainability is a wicked problem and that people can make decisions to act without trying to purify the problem into a simple dichotomy of "good" and "bad," without purifying it down to one, universal ideal, separate from society.

As we have seen from the historical case studies presented in Part I, ingestion as a metaphor for body-society relationships emerged in tandem with the idea of purity, freedom, sanitation, and science. Modern ideas of self, body, and society have been built around powerful material and conceptual boundaries and dichotomies. However, we are now at the point where these purification solutions are biting back, creating other risks—effects of our actions not intended or predicted, leading to conundrums and further attempts to control effects through further boundary making and purification treadmills.

Purity politics, Part II has shown, is a static and untenable way to deal with the problems we face today. Sustainable transformations will therefore require new metaphors. I am suggesting fermentation and digestion as promising possibilities. Fermentation opens up the world to the outside, but avoids the chaos of disorder. Chaotic fermentation just leads to a bigger mess. Good ferment requires good processes. Fermentation is therefore not a metaphor of anarchy but of governance, of founding new ways of collaborating. Digestion as a metaphor also reminds us of how we live after we have made our choices. How do we live with our decisions, our path dependencies, like suburban sprawl planning, conventional agriculture, nuclear power, wars for oil, or even something more annoying than destructive, such as noisy wind power projects?

Alternative ways of life, from a fermentive / digestive perspective, are not a romantic embrace of the outside as salvation but a collaborative engagement. Not surprisingly, agroecologists have shown a particular openness to this more transformational form of knowing. Faced with the issue of tacit vs. codified knowledge, agroecology has had to open itself up to society and nature in ways not experienced in more conventional sciences. Those who teach agroecology argue that the goal of teaching complex environmental and sustainability issues is to "open" the problems rather than solve them, in a process in which the teacher learns about the issue along with the students. A more inclusive teaching strategy, bringing students into the field or farmers into the classroom, is absolutely necessary for this kind of teaching. In their environmental studies courses, François Mélard and Nathalie Semal use a teaching process they refer to as "symmetry": an opportunity for students "to hesitate, i.e. to be confronted—even emotionally—to the unexpected, and the opportunity to come up with different ways of seeing the problem and different ways to make decisions."[10] Mélard and Semal use a pedagogy that confronts students with actors' different ways of thinking and presents environmental issues as diverging rather than converging toward consensus. From this perspective, professors facilitate new knowledge through mutual exploration based on different worldviews.

The contemporary case studies in Part II showed that today's world is full of conundrums but that the way we see our bodies in relation to the world is changing, and that these changes signal possible opportunities for a new politics. Alternative economies are powerful but not perfect. They are unfixed; that is, they are always open to question. It is this "unfixedness" that makes it necessary to keep food systems engaged in the larger, ongoing civic conversation about making a better world, with the "better" defined differently, reflexively, and collectively by different people. It is the process of building this world despite our different worldviews that makes the dynamics of alternative economies so complex and so powerful. Reflexivity is the political practice that can make the power of alternative economies manifest in a more inclusive and livable world. Reflexivity requires abandoning perfect politics and opening up Western social understanding beyond bounded good and bad behavior.

An imperfect politics of food is different from a safe food politics. But it is also not a *caveat emptor* politics. Instead, people can accept a world in which trade-offs and risks are unavoidable, and then can go about making the necessary but messy bargains about how they will share those risks. Often these bargains become embedded in institutions such as regulatory agencies. In a world of imperfect politics, there are no revelatory angels, no protective soldiers who represent the common good. Since we can't wall ourselves off from the risky world of untrustworthy actors and institutions and tricky bacteria, we need to work with them. So, we are left making bargains for our safety with those who will not make us fully safe. We are also tempted by those who tell us the opposite story: that the world is full of beings and institutions bent on our destruction, that we must abandon all and make the world anew. But complete faith in such a story will return us to the treadmill of purity. Trade-offs will not mean that all consequences are foreseeable, but at least some of the risks will be acknowledged ahead of time.

What would the agroecology of a food system look like, based on these processes? First, people would understand that our current fresh food system—such as milk and vegetables—depends on industrial organization. As Alfred Chandler tells us in his history of the modern economy, the fluid milk dairy system provided one of the first models of industrial organization. A consistent supply of fresh milk all year long is only possible through industrial processes and, in fact, is the first form of agriculture to develop confined animal feeding operations and large-scale distribution systems. Abandoning factory farming means trade-offs. An agroecological system would look more like the sign on my local organic grocery store shelf where the goats' milk yogurt usually sits: "Goats on Vacation: Less yogurt available until spring." If we truly want our dairy system to be pastoral, to maintain our small dairy farms on a landscape of open meadows, we have to abandon what the large-scale industrial milk system gives us: fresh milk, all year long. We can't just purify the system by setting grass-fed standards. We have to decide to make milk seasonal again, with a dairy price system that honors the nonfresh product as well, rather than something like pizza cheese becoming the garbage can for surplus milk that doesn't make it into the higher-priced fluid market. In particular, we have to admit that fresh raw milk all year long is a romantic dream. Fresh milk all year long is intrinsically based on an industrial system that requires large-scale science, government purification, and large-scale industrial organization. Collaborating with bacteria, and with seasons, along with honoring—with a better pricing system—the nonfresh product, may yield a more diverse dairy system that could lead to new hybridities and diversities. Wherever it led, it wouldn't be to more pizza cheese.

The relationship between the city and the country would also need to be renegotiated. It would not involve simply setting standards and imposing them on farmers. If commodities do mirror politics, then the new politics would lead to new foods, created by interactive processes in which consumers and producers—farmers and laborers—would negotiate what it is they could possibly grow and possibly eat. "Fair Trade" would not be a label but a process in which the definition of fairness was part of an ongoing and open civic conversation.[11] "Organic" would be a way of growing that involved partnerships in the risk of growing food, rather than a market niche that only a few have been able to successfully exploit, leaving the economy littered with the husks of failed organic farms. Organic food would mean food produced through organic processes, not just on the farm but all the way to the consumer. It would be a world made better because we let the world in, not because we kept it out.

Agroecology as a field of research and a relationship to nature provides an example of this new "post-normal" kind of knowing. It points to the ways in which science—that is, our ways of knowing the world—can become more open, "a social activity, both highly distributed and radically reflexive."[12] The role of science in society has already changed: "Science does not enter a chaotic society to put order into it any more, to simplify its composition, and to put an end to its controversies," states Bruno Latour. Instead, "when scientists add their findings to the mix, they do not put an end to politics, they add new ingredients to the collective process."[13]

Even in 1964 there was some suspicion that the Iron Curtain imaginary could eventually get everyone in trouble. In that year, Stanley Kubrick released the film *Dr. Strangelove,* a black comedy about how a military commander ordered a nuclear holocaust to protect his "precious bodily fluids." "It's incredibly obvious, isn't it?" the general explains to the officer played by Peter Sellers, as they barrel along toward full-scale nuclear war: "A foreign substance is introduced into our precious bodily fluids, without the knowledge of the individual, certainly without any choice." The idea of protecting the autonomous body and its ability to make its own choice, what the Founders believed would create a social order based on the Enlightenment idea of individual freedom, becomes, in the film, the cause of social annihilation. The "foreign substance" in this case is Communism, and the general protects his bodily fluids by defending the world from Communism and denying women his "bodily essence." The situation described in the film, that our protections are based on exclusions and that those exclusions in fact lead to greater risks, is a conundrum that we increasingly must face, as the risks of social annihilation multiply.

What this new, more inclusive sustainability politics would look like is still uncertain. We are currently faced with political conundrums about how to go about creating these collective processes, and our conversations about food reflect these conundrums. We need to find a new way to know and grow food, as a new way to understand ourselves and how we as bodies relate, politically, to the social world we inhabit. Perhaps fermentation as a metaphor will enable us to know these things differently, in a way that will allow us to better understand the political possibilities and potential choices we have—and don't have—for the future. Perhaps seeing our personal bodies as metabiomes will enable us to imagine the body of society in different ways so that we, as bodies, can relate to the world, and see how the world relates to us, differently. Maybe this new way of looking at the body will allow a certain abandonment of the treadmill of control and purification, of the maintenance of "bodily essence": relief from the idea of an intact self. But it will require good processes, new kinds of inclusive and just governance that we must build to create a better future.

NOTES

INTRODUCTION

1. Philip White, *Our Supreme Task: How Winston Churchill's Iron Curtain Speech Defined the Cold War Alliance* (New York: Public Affairs, 2012), 192.

2. Ibid., 187.

3. In Critical Theory, there is a long-standing conversation between those who claim bounding and bifurcation as a universal category, necessary for identity, and those who claim that narrating the world, and the self, through dualisms is a historically situated practice. The universalizers include psychoanalytic theorist Julia Kristeva, whose essay "The Powers of Horror" has been extremely influential in the conversation. Anne McClintock's *Imperial Leather*, Edward Said's *Orientalism*, and other works have situated cultural bifurcations specifically in the rise of modern Western culture. Works such as Paul Gilroy's *The Black Diaspora* represent ways of doing history that explicitly reject boundaries and bifurcations as intrinsic to historical narrative, emphasizing instead mixing and flows of culture. Doris Witt's *Black Hunger* and Kyla Wazana Tompkins's *Racial Indigestion* explicitly examine cultural confoundings of race and food, examining the history of food as associated with particular bodies. Finally, Donna Haraway's *Cyborg Manifesto*, which explores hybridity in Western culture, has greatly informed the conversation and this book.

4. Frederick Kaufman, *A Short History of the American Stomach* (Orlando: Houghton Mifflin Harcourt, 2008), xiv.

5. Ibid., *Short History*, xv.

6. "Biopolitics" is a term introduced into the contemporary literature by Michel Foucault in *Society Must Be Defended: Lectures at the Collège de France, 1975–76* (New York: Picador, 2003). "Gastropolitics" is a term first introduced by Arjun Appadurai in "Gastropolitics in Hindu South Asia," *American Ethnologist* 8 (1981): 494–511. See also Parama Roy, "Meat-Eating, Masculinity and Renunciation in India: A Gandhian Grammar of Diet," *Gender and History* 14, no. 1 (2002).

7. Julie Guthman and E. Melanie DuPuis, "Embodying Neoliberalism: Economy, Culture, and the Politics of Fat," *Environment and Planning D: Society and Space* 24, no. 3 (2006).

8. Andrew Pickering, "The Mangle of Practice: Agency and Emergence in the Sociology of Science," *American Journal of Sociology* 99, no. 3 (1993): 567.

9. Francesca Polletta, *It Was Like a Fever: Storytelling in Protest and Politics* (Chicago: University of Chicago Press, 2006).

10. Kyla Wazana Tompkins, *Racial Indigestion: Eating Bodies in the 19th Century* (New York: New York University Press, 2012), 3.

11. Ibid.

12. The psychoanalytical view of the relationship between body and society was originally laid out by Jacques Lacan and later rethought by feminist theorists Julia Kristeva and Judith Butler.

13. Interview with Susan Buck-Morss, "Sometimes to Progress Means to Stop, to Pull the Emergency Brake," *Kultura Liberalna* blog, December 27, 2011, accessed June 18, 2014, http://kulturaliberalna.pl/2011/12/27/sometimes-to-progress-means-to-stop-to-pull-the-emergency-brake/.

14. http://globalization.gc.cuny.edu/2012/01/susan-buck-morss-sometimes-to-progress-means-to-stop-to-pull-the-emergency-brake/.

15. David Morely and Kuan-Sing Chen, eds., *Stuart Hall: Critical Dialogues in Cultural Studies* (New York: Routledge, 1996), 444.

16. Peter Vandergeest, "Real Villages: National Narratives of Rural Development," in *Creating the Countryside: The Politics of Rural and Environmental Discourse,* ed. E. Melanie DuPuis and Peter Vandergeest (Philadelphia: Temple University Press, 1996).

17. Mary Douglas, *Purity and Danger: An Analysis of Concepts of Pollution and Taboo* (New York: Praeger, 1966); Bruno Latour, *The Pasteurization of France* (Cambridge, MA: Harvard University Press, 1988).

18. Tompkins, *Racial Indigestion.*

CHAPTER I: FREE AND ORDERLY BODIES

1. Gordon S. Wood, *Empire of Liberty: A History of the Early Republic, 1789–1815* (New York: Oxford University Press, 2009), 41.

2. Lynn Hunt, *Inventing Human Rights: A History* (New York: W. W. Norton, 2008), 29.

3. John Coveney, *Food, Morals and Meaning: The Pleasures and Anxiety of Eating* (New York: Routledge, 2000), 8.

4. David Brion Davis, *The Problem of Slavery in the Age of Revolution* (New York: Oxford University Press, 1999), 7.

5. Ibid., 4.

6. Hunt, *Inventing Human Rights,* 29.

7. Davis, *Problem of Slavery,* 263.

8. Ibid.

9. Richard Hofstadter, *The American Political Tradition and the Men Who Made It* (New York: Random House, 1967), 13.

10. James Madison, *Federalist Papers,* #51.

11. Ibid.

12. Wood, *Empire of Liberty.*

13. John Adams, *Novanglus Letters, No. III* (1774); Andrew S. Trees, *The Founding Fathers and the Politics of Character* (Princeton, NJ: Princeton University Press, 2003).

14. Edmund S. Morgan, "Slavery and Freedom: The American Paradox," *Journal of American History* 59, no. 1 (1972): 5–29.

15. Eric Foner, *Free Soil, Free Labor, Free Men: The Ideology of the Republican Party Before the Civil War* (New York: Oxford University Press, 1995).

16. Dagobert D. Runes, ed., *The Selected Writings of Benjamin Rush* (New York: Philosophical Library, 2007), 168.

17. Noga Arikha, *Passions and Tempers: A History of the Humours* (New York: Ecco, 2007), 99.

18. Rush quoted in Donald J. D'Elia, "Benjamin Rush: Philosopher of the American Revolution," *Transaction of the American Philosophical Society* 64, no. 5 (1974): 68.

19. D'Elia, "Benjamin Rush," 68.

20. Runes, *Selected Writings of Benjamin Rush,* 209.

21. Ibid., 193.

22. Alyn Brodsky, *Benjamin Rush: Patriot and Physician* (New York: Truman Talley, 2004), 96.

23. Wood, *Empire of Liberty,* 43–44.

24. Letter from Benjamin Rush to John Adams, June 13, 1808, in *Our Sacred Honor: Words of Advice from the Founders in Stories, Letters, Poems, and Speeches,* ed. William John Bennett (New York: Simon & Schuster, 1997), 89.

25. Several of these appear at the end of Benjamin Rush, *Essays: Literary, Moral and Philosophical* (Philadelphia: University of Pennsylvania, 1798).

26. Benjamin Rush, *Enquiry into the Effects of Spirituous Liquors on the Human Body,* Early American Imprints, 1st series, no. 22864, 1790.

27. L. H. Butterfield, ed., *Letters of Benjamin Rush* (Princeton, NJ: Princeton University Press, 1951).

28. James Henry Morgan, *Dickinson College: A History of One Hundred and Fifty Years, 1783–1933.* Dickinson College webpage, accessed January 17, 2015, http://chronicles.dickinson.edu/histories/morgan/chapter_3.html.

29. François Furstenberg, "Beyond Freedom and Slavery: Autonomy, Virtue, and Resistance in Early American Political Discourse," *Journal of American History* 89, no. 4 (2003): 1309.

30. The Jefferson Monticello website, accessed March, 28, 2015, www.monticello.org/site/jefferson/dinner-served.

31. Furstenberg, "Beyond Freedom and Slavery."

1. Ralph Waldo Emerson, "New England Reformers," in *The Selected Writings of Ralph Waldo Emerson*, ed. Brooks Atkinson (New York: Modern Library, 1950), 449–50.

2. Emerson, "New England Reformers."

3. Aidan Day, *Romanticism: The New Critical Idiom* (London and New York: Routledge Taylor & Francis Group, 2012).

4. John L. Thomas, "Romantic Reform in America, 1815–1865," *American Quarterly* 17, no. 4 (Winter 1965): 657.

5. Alexis de Tocqueville, *Democracy in America*, Penn State Electronic Classics Series Publication (University Park: Penn State University Press, 2002 [1835]), 610.

6. David S. Reynolds, *Waking Giant: America in the Age of Jackson* (New York: Harper Perennial, 2008), 238.

7. Ibid., 112.

8. Ibid., 661.

9. Eric Foner, *Free Soil, Free Labor, Free Men: The Ideology of the Republican Party before the Civil War* (New York: Oxford University Press, 1995), 924.

10. Jane H. Pease and William H. Pease, "Confrontation and Abolition in the 1850s," *Journal of American History* 58, no. 4 (1972): 923–24.

11. Thomas, "Romantic Reform in America," 661.

12. Emerson, "New England Reformers," 449.

13. Walter Stahr, *Seward: Lincoln's Indispensable Man* (New York: Simon & Schuster, 2012).

14. Edwin H. Ford and Edwin Emery, *Highlights in the History of the American Press: A Book of Readings* (Minneapolis: University of Minnesota Press, 1954), 137.

15. Thomas C. Leonard, *Power of the Press : The Birth of American Political Reporting* (Cary, NC: Oxford University Press, 1986), 86.

16. Thomas R. Pegram, *Battling Demon Rum: The Struggle for a Dry America* (Chicago: Ivan R. Dee, 1998).

17. Foner, *Free Soil, Free Labor, Free Men*, xiii.

18. Ibid.

19. Ibid., xi.

20. Ibid.

21. Ibid.

22. Reynolds, *Waking Giant*.

23. William Lloyd Garrison, "American Slavery: Address on the Subject of American Slavery, and the Progress of the Cause of Freedom throughout the World," speech delivered September 2, 1846, accessed January 17, 2015, http://find.galegroup .com.oca.ucsc.edu/mome/infomark.

24. Susan Schulten, "A Capitalist Case for Emancipation," *Opinionator, New York Times,* accessed February 6, 2013, http://opinionator.blogs.nytimes.com /2013/02/06/a-capitalist-case-for-emancipation/.

25. Ibid.

26. Michelle C. Neely, "Embodied Politics: Antebellum Vegetarianism and the Dietary Economy of *Walden*," *American Literature* 85, no. 1 (2013).

27. Sylvester Graham, *Lectures on the Science of Human Life* (London: Boston, Marsh, Capen, Lyon & Webb, 1849), 112.

28. Ralph Waldo Emerson, "Man the Reformer," in *Essays and Poems of Emerson* (New York: Harcourt Brace, 1921), 317.

29. Adam D. Shprintzen, *Vegetarian Crusade: The Rise of an American Reform Movement, 1817–1921* (Chapel Hill: University of North Carolina Press, 2013), 113.

30. Ibid., 113. Greeley's paper had called upon the Union Army to move "Forward to Richmond" to finish the Civil War quickly. Prompted in part by the *Tribune's* call, the Union suffered great losses at Bull Run. Many readers rushed to unsubscribe and the *Herald* rushed to attack.

31. Ibid., 113.

32. *Herald* newspaper articles quoted in Shprintzen, *Vegetarian Crusade,* 112, 113.

33. Ronald L. Numbers, *Prophetess of Health: Ellen G. White and the Origins of Seventh-Day Adventist Health Reform* (Knoxville: University of Tennessee Press, 1992).

34. Thomas, "Romantic Reform in America," 658.

35. Ibid., 656.

36. Richard Lyman Bushman, *Joseph Smith: Rough Stone Rolling* (New York: Alfred A. Knopf, 2005).

37. Gilbert Seldes, *The Stammering Century* (New York: NYRB Classics, 2012), 119.

38. Chas. H. Barfoot, *Aimee Semple McPherson and the Making of Modern Pentecostalism, 1890–1926* (New York: Routledge, 2014).

39. Numbers, *Prophetess of Health.*

40. "Vegetarianism," *Oxford Encyclopedia of Food and Drink in America* (New York: Oxford University Press, 2004).

41. Priscilla J. Brewer, "The Demographic Features of the Shaker Decline, 1787–1900," *Journal of Interdisciplinary History* 15 (1984).

42. E. Melanie DuPuis, *Nature's Perfect Food: How Milk Became America's Drink* (New York: NYU Press, 2002).

43. Isaac Smithson Hartley, *Memorial of Robert Milham Hartley* (New York: Arno Press, 1976).

44. Quoted in Shprintzen, 28.

45. William Lloyd Garrison, "The War: Its Cause and Its Cure," *The Liberator,* May 3, 1861.

46. Blake McKelvey, "Flour Milling at Rochester," *Rochester History* 33 (1971).

47. How Graham, who was so wrong about the evils of spices and masturbation, managed to figure out that milling the bran out of flour made it less nutritious is unclear.

48. Michael B. Katz, Michael K. Doucet, and Mark Stern, *The Social Organization of Early Industrial Capitalism* (Cambridge, MA: Harvard University Press, 1982), 29.

49. Ibid.

50. Regarding the idea that certain social classes create their status through "self-fashioning," see Steven Jay Greenblatt, *Renaissance Self-Fashioning: From More to Shakespeare* (Chicago: University of Chicago Press, 1980).

51. Joseph R. Gusfield, *Symbolic Crusade: Status Politics and the American Temperance Movement* (Champaign: University of Illinois Press, 1986).

52. Judith N. MacArthur, "Demon Rum on the Boards: Temperance Melodrama and the Tradition of Antebellum Reform," *Journal of the Early Republic* 9 (1989); James L. McElroy, "Social Control and Romantic Reform in Antebellum America: The Case of Rochester, New York," *New York History* 58 (1977); Paul E. Johnson, *A Shopkeeper's Millenium: Society and Revivals in Rochester, NY, 1815–1837* (New York: Hill and Wang, 1978); Whitney Cross, *The Burned-Over District: The Social and Intellectual History of Enthusiastic Religion in Western New York, 1800–1850* (New York: Octagon, 1981).

53. E. Melanie DuPuis, "Angels and Vegetables: A Brief History of Food Advice in America," *Gastronomica: The Journal of Food and Culture* 7, no. 3 (Summer 2007): 34–44. McArthur, "Demon Rum on the Boards," 528.

54. Lance Newman, "Sullen Fires across the Atlantic: Essays in Transatlantic Romanticism," *Romantic Circles: A Refereed Scholarly Website Devoted to the Study of Romantic-period Literature and Culture,* accessed January 18, 2015, www.rc.umd.edu/praxis/sullenfires/intro/intro.html.

55. Timothy Morton, "Joseph Ritson, Percy Shelley and the Making of Romantic Vegetarianism," *Romanticism* 12, no. 1 (2006): 58, 59.

56. Graham, *Lectures on the Science of Human Life,* 6.

57. Shprintzen, *Vegetarian Crusade,* 27.

58. Ibid., 25.

59. Ibid., 22.

60. Ibid.

61. Ibid.

62. Lawrence W. Levine, *Highbrow / Lowbrow: The Emergence of Cultural Hierarchy in America* (Cambridge, MA: Harvard University Press, 1988), 140.

63. Joel Pace, "Towards a Taxonomy of Transatlantic Romanticism(s)," *Literature Compass* 5, no. 2 (2008): 256.

64. Amanda Claybaugh, "Toward a New Transatlanticism: Dickens in the United States," *Victorian Studies* 8, no. 3 (2006): 439.

65. Edward Pessen, "How Different from Each Other Were the Antebellum North and South," *American Historical Review* 85 (1980): 1139.

66. Drew Gilpin Faust, "A Southern Stewardship: The Intellectual and the Proslavery Argument," *American Quarterly* 31, no. 1 (1979): 68.

67. Ibid.

68. Gusfield, *Symbolic Crusade.*

69. William R. Taylor, *Cavalier and Yankee: The Old South and American National Character* (New York: Oxford University Press, 1993).

70. Ibid., 96.

71. Ibid., 123.

72. Joe Gray Taylor, *Eating, Drinking and Visiting in the South: An Informal History* (Baton Rouge: Louisiana State University Press, 1982), 91.

73. Mary Titus, "The Dining Room Door Swings Both Ways: Food, Race and Domestic Space in the Nineteenth Century South," in *Haunted Bodies: Gender and Southern Texts,* ed. Anne Goodwyn Jones and Susan V. Donaldson (Charlottesville: University Press of Virginia, 1997), 243.

74. Taylor, *Eating, Drinking and Visiting in the South.*

75. Mary Randolph, *The Virginia Housewife, or Methodical Cook* (Baltimore: Plaskit Fite, 1838), 12.

76. Kyla Wazana Tompkins, *Racial Indigestion: Eating Bodies in the 19th Century* (New York: New York University Press, 2012).

77. Elizabeth Fox Genovese, *Within the Plantation Household: Black and White Women of the Old South* (Chapel Hill: University of North Carolina Press, 1988), 98.

78. Mary Boykin Chesnut, *The Private Mary Chesnut: The Unpublished Civil War Diaries* (New York: Oxford University Press, 1984), 73.

79. Taylor, *Cavalier and Yankee,* 157.

80. Ibid., 285.

81. Judith N. McArthur, "Demon Rum on the Boards: Temperance Melodrama and the Tradition of Antebellum Reform," *Journal of the Early Republic* 9, no. 4 (Winter 1989).

82. Pessen, "How Different from Each Other," 1124.

83. Foner, *Free Soil, Free Labor, Free Men,* 9.

84. Reynolds, *Waking Giant.*

85. Ibid.

86. Charles Lane and Bronson Alcott, "The Consociate Family Life," *Liberator* 13 (1843): 152.

87. Thomas, "Romantic Reform in America."

88. Emerson diary, unclear date, sometime in November 1842.

89. Louisa May Alcott, *Transcendental Wild Oats and Excerpts from the Fruitlands Diary* (Harvard, MA: Harvard Common Press, 1981). Also in Clara Endicott Sears, ed., *Bronson Alcott's Fruitlands with Transcendental Wild Oats, by Louisa M. Alcott* (Boston: Houghton Mifflin, 1915).

90. John Farina, ed., *Isaac T. Hecker, The Diary: Romantic Religion in Antebellum America* (New York: Paulist Press, 1988).

91. T. Gregory Garvey, *Creating the Culture of Reform in Antebellum America* (Athens: University of Georgia Press, 2006), 138.

92. Shprintzen, *Vegetarian Crusade.*

93. Garvey, *Creating the Culture of Reform,* 5 (emphasis mine).

1. Sidney Pollard, "Factory Discipline in the Industrial Revolution," *Economic History Review* 16, no. 2 (1963); Herbert G. Gutman, "Work, Culture, and Society in Industrializing America," *American Historical Review* (1973).

2. Richard Edwards, *Contested Terrain* (New York: Basic Books, 1980).

3. This verse is from the song "Many Thousands Gone."

4. Herbert C. Covey and Dwight Eisnach, *What the Slaves Ate: Recollections of African American Foods and Foodways from the Slave Narratives* (Santa Barbara, CA: ABC-CLIO, 2009).

5. Psyche A. Williams-Forson, *Building Houses Out of Chicken Legs: Black Women, Food, and Power* (Chapel Hill: University of North Carolina Press, 2006).

6. Elizabeth Brabec and Sharon Richardson, "A Clash of Cultures: The Landscape of the Sea Island Gullah," *Landscape Journal* 26 (2007): 1–7.

7. Rufus B. Saxton, quoted in Edwin D. Hoffman, "From Slavery to Self-Reliance: The Record of Achievement of the Freedmen of the Sea Island Region," *Journal of Negro History* 41 (1956): 9.

8. Charles Spencer, *Edisto Island, 1861 to 2006: Ruin, Recovery and Rebirth* (Charleston, SC: History Press, 2008).

9. Richard H. Abbott, *Cotton and Capital: Boston Businessmen and Antislavery Reform, 1854–1868* (Amherst: University of Massachusetts Press, 1991), 86

10. Hoffman, "From Slavery to Self-Reliance," 9.

11. Ibid., 16.

12. Williams-Forson, *Building Houses Out of Chicken Legs.*

13. Rachel Naomi Klein, "Harriet Beecher Stowe and the Domestication of Free Labor Ideology," *Legacy* 18, no. 2 (2001): 137.

14. Ibid., 138.

15. Eric Foner and Olivia Mahoney, *America's Reconstruction: People and Politics after the Civil War* (Baton Rouge: Louisiana State University Press, 1997), 15.

16. George Howe Colt, *The Big House: A Century of Life in an American Summer Home* (New York: Scribner, 2004), 22.

17. Saxton, quoted in Hoffman, "From Slavery to Self-Reliance," 16. And the fact that the ginning occurred in the North meant that the seeds for next year's cotton harvest were lost, one of the reasons contributing to the decline of Sea Islands cotton after the war.

18. Hoffman, "From Slavery to Self-Reliance," 21.

19. Lawrence N. Powell, *New Masters: Northern Planters during the Civil War and Reconstruction* (New Haven, CT: Yale University Press, 1980).

20. Richard H. Abbott, "A Yankee Views the Organization of the Republican Party in South Carolina, July 1867," *South Carolina Historical Magazine* 85, no. 3 (1984): 245.

21. Sea Islands freedmen, who became known as the Gullah, fought continually for land access and to maintain a vegetable and corn agriculture. In fact, by 1870,

much of the Sea Islands region was owned by African Americans, eventually becoming a vegetable truck-farming area. Particularly with the ravages of the boll weevil, but also through agroecological struggles, Sea Islands cotton agriculture has disappeared into the past, replaced by small black agricultural communities of vegetable and subsistence growers—flanked by resort motels. In this case, the struggle to control one's diet was not the product of Northern dietary advice but the freedom to create a new local agroecology around a particular autonomous diet. For a description see Brabec and Richardson, "Clash of Cultures," 1–7.

22. Rufus B. Saxton to E. S. Philbrick, Rufus B. and S. Willard Saxton Papers, Manuscripts and Archives, Yale University Library, Low Country Digital History Archives, accessed July 30, 2014, http://ldhi.library.cofc.edu/exhibits/show /after_slavery_educator/unit_three_documents/document four.

23. Klein, "Harriet Beecher Stowe."

24. Stowe quoted in Powell, *New Masters,* 111.

25. Ibid.

26. Sam Bowers Hilliard, *Hog Meat and Hoecake: Food Supply in the Old South, 1840–1860* (Carbondale: Southern Illinois University Press), 67.

27. Eric Foner, *Politics and Ideology in the Age of the Civil War* (New York: Oxford University Press, 1980), 150

28. Zora Neale Hurston, *Their Eyes Were Watching God* (New York: HarperCollins, 1999).

29. Carolyn Finney, *Black Faces, White Spaces: Reimagining the Relationship of African Americans to the Great Outdoors* (Chapel Hill: University of North Carolina Press, 2014), 55.

30. Catharine Beecher and Harriet Beecher Stowe, *The American Woman's Home: Principles of Domestic Science* (Carlisle, MA: Applewood Books, 2008), 458.

31. Powell, *New Masters.*

32. Tourgeé quoted in Natalie J. Ring, *The Problem South: Region, Empire and the New Liberal State, 1880–1930* (Athens: University of Georgia, 2012), 28.

33. Ibid., 31.

34. Beecher quoted in Powell, *New Masters,* 262.

35. Juliet Corson, *Cooking School Text Book; and Housekeepers' Guide to Cookery and Kitchen Management* (New York: O. Judd, 1883).

36. E. Melaine DuPuis, *Nature's Perfect Food: How Milk Became America's Drink* (New York: New York University Press, 2002).

37. Laura Shapiro, *Perfection Salad* (New York: Random House, 2001).

38. Ibid., 88.

39. Hasia R. Diner, *Hungering for America: Italian, Irish and Jewish Foodways in the Age of Migration* (Cambridge, MA: Harvard University Press, 2001), xvii.

40. Maureen Ogle, *In Meat We Trust: An Unexpected History of Carnivore America* (Boston: Houghton Mifflin, 2013), front flap.

41. Ibid., 12.

42. K. Dun Gifford, "Dietary Fats, Eating Guides, and Public Policy: History, Critique, and Recommendations," *American Journal of Medicine* 113, no. 9 (2002).

43. W. O. Atwater, "A Pecuniary Economy of Food: The Chemistry of Food and Nutrition," *The Century: A Popular Quarterly* 35, no. 3 (1888). 437.

44. Ellen Swallow Richards, "Preface," in Mary Hinman Abel, *The Rumford Kitchen Leaflets: No. 17, The Story of the New England Kitchen; Part II, A Study in Social Economics* (Boston: Home Science, 1899), 132.

45. Harvey Levenstein, *Revolution at the Table: The Transformation of the American Diet* (Berkeley: University of California Press, 2003).

46. Ibid.

47. Atwater relied on the calorimeter, a closed room that calculated the calories expended by a worker by measuring his respiration.

48. W. O. Atwater, "What We Should Eat," *The Century: A Popular Quarterly* 36 (1888): 257.

49. Charlotte Biltekoff, *Eating Right in America: The Cultural Politics of Food and Health* (Durham, NC: Duke University Press Books, 2013).

50. Samuel Gompers and Herman Gutstadt, *Meat vs. Rice: American Manhood against Asiatic Coolieism—Which Shall Survive?* (San Francisco: American Federation of Labor, 1901).

51. *Current Literature* 2, no. 2 (February 1889): 162.

52. Testimony to Senate Committee on Chinese Immigration, 1876, quoted in Almaguer (see note 53), 167.

53. Tomás Almaguer, *Racial Fault Lines: The Historical Origins of White Supremacy in California* (Berkeley: University of California Press, 2008).

54. Ibid., 164.

55. Eugene V. Debs, *Letters of Eugene V. Debs,* ed. J. Robert Constantine, vol. 1 (Champaign: University of Illinois Press, 1990), 41.

56. Gompers and Gustadt, *Meat vs. Rice,* 17.

57. Natalia Molina, *Fit to Be Citizens?: Public Health and Race in Los Angeles, 1879–1939* (Berkeley: University of California Press, 2006).

58. Gompers and Gutstadt, *Meat vs. Rice,* 14.

59. Arthur Schlesinger, "A Dietary Interpretation of American History," *Proceedings of the Massachusetts Historical Society* 3, no. 68 (1947): 207–8.

60. Harvey Levenstein, *A Paradox of Plenty: A Social History of Eating in Modern America* (Berkeley: University of California Press, 1994).

61. Ibid., 56–57.

62. Biltekoff, *Eating Right in America,* 28.

63. Michaela Sullivan-Fowler, "Doubtful Theories, Drastic Therapies: Autointoxication and Faddism in the Late Nineteenth and Early Twentieth Centuries," *Journal of the History of Medicine and Allied Sciences* 50 (1995).

64. Mark Pendergrast, *Uncommon Grounds: The History of Coffee and How It Transformed Our World* (New York: Basic Books, 2010).

1. Herbert Spencer, *The Man versus the State, with Six Essays on Government, Society and Freedom,* ed. Eric Mack, introduction by Albert Jay Nock (Indianapolis: LibertyClassics, 1981), accessed May 3, 2015, http://oll.libertyfund.org/titles/330, 396.

2. Charles McCann, *Order and Control in American Socio-Economic Thought: Social Scientists and Progressive-Era Reform* (London and New York: Routledge, 2012), 26.

3. Richard Hofstadter, *The Progressive Movement, 1900–1915* (Upper Saddle River, NJ: Prentice-Hall, 1963).

4. Robert H. Wiebe, *The Search for Order, 1877–1920* (New York: Hill and Wang, 1966).

5. Ibid., 128–29.

6. Ibid., 160.

7. Alain Corbin, *The Foul and the Fragrant: Odor and the French Social Imagination* (Cambridge, MA: Harvard University Press, 1986).

8. Nancy Tomes, *The Gospel of Germs: Men, Women, and the Microbe in American Life* (Cambridge, MA: Harvard University Press, 1998).

9. E. Melanie DuPuis, "Angels and Vegetables: A Brief History of Food Advice in America," *Gastronomica: The Journal of Critical Food Studies* 7, no. 3 (2007).

10. Tomes, *Gospel of Germs,* 34.

11. Priscilla Wald, Nancy Tomes, and Lisa Lynch, "Introduction: Culture and Contagion," Special Issue, *American Literary History* 14, no. 4 (Winter 2002): 219.

12. Kristen R. Egan, "Conservation and Cleanliness: Racial and Environmental Purity in Ellen Richards and Charlotte Perkins Gilman," *WSQ: Women's Studies Quarterly* 39, no. 3 (2011): 87.

13. Ibid., 87.

14. Hofstader, *Progressive Movement,* 218.

15. Ibid., 231.

16. McCann, *Order and Control,* 19.

17. Martha H. Verbrugge, *Able-Bodied Womanhood: Personal Health and Social Change in Nineteenth-Century Boston* (New York: Oxford University Press, 1988), 133.

18. Ibid., 135.

19. Hofstader, *Progressive Movement,* 236.

20. Roosevelt quoted in Hofstader, *Progressive Movement,* 237.

21. James Whorton, *Inner Hygiene: Constipation and the Pursuit of Health in Modern Society* (New York: Oxford University Press, 2003).

22. Marc Law and Gary D. Libecap, *The Determinants of Progressive Era Reform: The Pure Food and Drugs Act of 1906* (Chicago: University of Chicago Press, 2004).

23. Ellen Swallow Richards, *Euthenics, the Science of Controllable Environment: A Plea for Better Living Conditions as a First Step toward Higher Human Efficiency* (Boston: Whitcomb & Barrows, 1910), 7.

24. Sarah Stage and Virginia Bramble Vincenti, eds., *Rethinking Home Economics: Women and the History of a Profession* (Ithaca, NY: Cornell University Press, 1997), 24, 28.

25. Marilyn Gittell and Teresa Shtob, "Changing Women's Roles in Political Volunteerism and Reform of the City," *Signs* 5, no. 3 (1980): S67–S78

26. Clayton A. Coppin and Jack C. High, *The Politics of Purity: Harvey Washington Wiley and the Origins of Federal Food Policy* (Ann Arbor: University of Michigan Press, 1999).

27. Robert W. Dimand, "Irving Fisher and Modern Macroeconomics," *American Economic Review* 87, no. 2 (1997).

28. Robert W. Dimand and John Geanakoplos, "Celebrating Irving Fisher: The Legacy of a Great Economist," *American Journal of Economics and Sociology* 64, no. 1 (2005).

29. Whorton, *Inner Hygiene*, 69.

30. Egan, "Conservation and Cleanliness."

31. Alfred I. Tauber, *The Immune Self: Theory or Metaphor?* (New York: Cambridge University Press, 1994).

32. Whorton, *Inner Hygiene*.

33. Ibid.

34. Danone Institute, "Historical Commitment of the Danone Institute to Health," n.d., accessed September 10, 2008, www.danoneinstitute.org/about_danone_institute/history.php.

35. Francis Galton, *Inquiries into Human Faculty and Its Development* (New York: Macmillan, 1883), 25n.

36. Ibid, 25n.

37. For a history of the concept of "Race Suicide" see, for example, Miriam King and Steven Ruggles, "American Immigration, Fertility, and Race Suicide at the Turn of the Century," *Journal of Interdisciplinary History* 20, no. 3 (1990). Thomas C. Leonard, "Retrospectives: Eugenics and Economics in the Progressive Era," *Journal of Economic Perspectives* 19, no. 4 (2005).

38. *Carrie Buck v. John Hendren Bell,* Superintendent of State Colony for Epileptics and Feeble Minded, 274 U.S. 200, 47 S. Ct. 584, 71 L. Ed. 1000, 1927.

39. Martin S. Pernick, "Eugenics and Public Health in American History," *American Journal of Public Health* 87, no. 11 (1997): 1767.

40. Egan, "Conservation and Cleanliness," 82.

41. James Harvey Young, *Pure Food: Securing the Federal Food and Drugs Act of 1906* (Princeton, NJ: Princeton University Press, 1989), 293.

42. Edward J. Larson, *Sex, Race, and Science: Eugenics in the Deep South* (Baltimore: Johns Hopkins University Press, 1996), 52.

43. Harvey Young, *Pure Food,* 292–93.

44. League of Nations Mixed Committee on Nutrition, *Nutrition: Final Report of the Mixed Committee of the League of Nations on the Relation of Nutrition to Health, Agriculture, and Economic Policy* (Geneva 1937).

45. Cynthia Brantley, *Feeding Families: African Realities and British Ideas of Nutrition and Development in Early Colonial Africa* (Portsmouth, NH: Heinemann, 2002).

46. These cross-national comparisons were published in a 1936 multivolume report by the League of Nations Mixed Committee on Nutrition: "Report on the Physiological Bases of Nutrition."

47. Cynthia Brantley, "Kikiyu-Maasai Nutrition and Colonial Science: The Orr and Gilks Study in the Late 1920s Revisited," *International Journal of African Historical Studies* 30 (1997): 51.

48. For an analysis of Asian colonial subjects and masculinity, see Mrinalini Sinha, *Colonial Masculinity: The "Manly Englishman" and the "Effeminate Bengali" in the Late Nineteenth Century* (New York: Manchester University Press, 1995).

49. David Arnold, "British India and the "Beriberi Problem," 1798–1942," *Medical History* 54, no. 3 (2010).

50. Anon., "The Non-Beef-Eating Nations," *Saturday Evening Post,* November 13, 1869, 8.

51. T. Swann Harding, "Diet and Disease," *Scientific Monthly* 26, no. 2 (1928): 153.

52. For an analysis of Asian colonial subjects and masculinity, see Sinha, *Colonial Masculinity.*

53. Helen Zoe Viet, *Modern Food, Moral Food: Self-Control, Science and the Rise of Modern American Eating in the Early Twentieth Century* (Chapel Hill: University of North Carolina Press, 2013), 4.

54. John L. Buck, *Chinese Farm Economy* (Chicago: University of Chicago Press, 1930).

55. Frederick W. Mote in K. C. Chang, *Food in Chinese Culture: Anthropological and Historical Perspectives* (New Haven, CT: Yale University Press, 1977), 198, 201.

56. Eugene N. Anderson, *The Food of China* (New Haven, CT: Yale University Press, 1988), 125.

57. Mike Davis, *Late Victorian Holocausts: El Niño Famines and the Making of the Third World* (New York: Verso, 2002).

58. Elmer Verner McCollum, *The Newer Knowledge of Nutrition: The Use of Food for the Preservation of Vitality and Health* (New York: McMillan, 1918), 151.

59. Ibid., 151.

60. Elmer Verner McCollum, "Lamplighter in Public and Professional Understanding of Nutrition," *Agricultural History* 54, no. 1 (1980).

61. E. Melanie DuPuis, *Nature's Perfect Food: How Milk Became America's Drink* (New York: New York University Press, 2002).

62. Ibid.

63. Harvey Levenstein, *A Paradox of Plenty: A Social History of Eating in Modern America* (Berkeley: University of California Press, 1994).

64. Verner McCollum, *Newer Knowledge of Nutrition.*

65. Shapiro, *Perfection Salad,* 90–91.

66. Ulysses P. Hedrick, *History of Agriculture in the State of New York* (Albany: New York State Agriculture Society, 1933).

67. Gerald V. O'Brien, "Indigestible Foods, Conquering Hordes and Waste Materials: Metaphors of Immigrants and the Early Immigration Restriction Debate in the United States," *Metaphor and Symbol* 18 (2003): 36–37.

68. Susan Currell and Christina Cogdell, *Popular Eugenics: National Efficiency and American Mass Culture in the 1930s* (Athens: Ohio University Press, 2006).

69. DuPuis, *Nature's Perfect Food.*

CHAPTER 5: GOOD FOOD, BAD ROMANCE

1. The latest trend data is from 2009: Centers for Disease Control, "State-Specific Trends in Fruit and Vegetable Consumption among Adults—United States, 2000–2009," *Morbidity and Mortality Weekly Report* 59, no. 5 (2010), accessed December 30, 2014, www.cdc.gov/mmwr/pdf/wk/mm5935.pdf.

2. Quoted in Sharon Begley, "Obesity Fight Must Shift from Personal Blame—US Panel," *Reuters,* US edition, May 8, 2012, accessed December 28, 2014, www.reuters.com/article/2012/05/08/us-usa-health-obesity.

3. Barry M. Popkin, "The Nutrition Transition and Obesity in the Developing World," *American Society for Nutritional Sciences* 131, no. 3 (2001); Barry M. Popkin and Colleen M. Doak, "The Obesity Epidemic Is a Worldwide Phenomenon," *Nutrition Reviews* 56, no. 4 (1998).

4. A.H. Mokdad et al., "Prevalence of Obesity, Diabetes, and Obesity-related Health Risk Factors," *Journal of the American Medical Association* 289, no. 1 (2003).

5. Popkin, "Nutrition Transition and Obesity."

6. Jean Baudrillard, *America* (New York: Verso, 1988). 76.

7. Michael Pollan, *The Omnivore's Dilemma: A Natural History of Four Meals* (New York: Penguin, 2006); Eric Schlosser, *Fast Food Nation: The Dark Side of the All-American Meal* (New York: Houghton Mifflin, 2001).

8. Tim Lang and Michael Heasman, *Food Wars: The Global Battle for Mouths, Minds and Markets* (London: Earthscan, 2004), 11.

9. Ibid., 13.

10. Ted Genoways, " 'I felt like a piece of trash'—Life inside America's Food Processing Plants," *The Guardian,* December 20, 2014, accessed December 30, 2014, www.theguardian.com/world/2014/dec/21/life-inside-america-food-processing-plants-cheap-meat.

11. *Science Daily,* "Quality of U.S. Diet Improves, Gap Widens for Quality between Rich and Poor," September 1, 2014, accessed December 30, 2014, www.sciencedaily.com/releases/2014/09/140901211535.htm.

12. Sylvester Graham, *Lectures on the Science of Human Life* (London: Boston, Marsh, Capen, Lyon & Webb, 1849), 112.

13. Barbara Kingsolver, Camille Kingsolver, and Steven L Hopp, *Animal, Vegetable, Miracle: A Year of Food Life* (New York: Harper Perennial, 2008), 3.

14. Ibid., 8.

15. Amy Cotler, *The Locavore Way: Discover and Enjoy the Pleasures of Locally Grown Food* (North Adams, MA: Storey, 2009), 1.

16. Ashima Kant and Barry Graubard, "Eating Out in America, 1987–2000: Trends and Nutritional Correlates," *Preventive Medicine* 38, no. 2 (2004): 243.

17. Julie Guthman, "Bringing Good Food to Others: Investigating the Subjects of Alternative Food Practice," *Cultural Geographies* 15, no. 4 (2008).

18. Kingsolver, et al., 8; Wendell Berry, "The Pleasures of Eating," in *Bringing It to the Table: On Farming and Food* (Berkeley: Counterpoint Press, 2009), 228.

19. Guthman, "Bringing Good Food to Others," 211.

20. NPR, "Alice Waters: 40 Years of Sustainable Food," August 27, 2011, accessed December 31, 2014, www.npr.org/2011/08/22/139707078/alice-waters-40-years-of-sustainable-food.

21. Marie Sarita Gaytán, "Globalizing Resistance: Slow Food and New Local Imaginaries," *Food, Culture and Society: An International Journal of Multidisciplinary Research* 7, no. 2 (2004): 108.

22. Ibid., 112.

23. Deborah Madison, "Forward," in *Slow Food: Collected Thoughts on Taste, Traditions and the Honest Pleasures of Food,* ed. C. Petrini and B. Watson (White River Junction, VT: Chelsea Green, 2001), ix.

24. Publicity blurb on Amazon website for book, *French Women Don't Get Fat,* accessed December 28, 2014, www.amazon.com/French-Women-Dont-Get-Fat/dp/0375710515.

25. Marie Savard on *Good Morning America,* June 24, 2009, video accessed December 31, 2014, http://abcnews.go.com/video/playerIndex?id = 7915630.

26. See, for example, "Mediterranean Diet Plan vs. American Diet Plan," Livestrong.com website, accessed December 31, 2014, www.livestrong.com/article/239583-mediterranean-diet-plan-vs-american-diet-plan/.

27. Dan Childs, "Take It or Leave It? The Truth About 8 Mediterranean Diet Staples," ABCNews online, June 24, 2009, accessed December 31, 2014, http://abcnews.go.com/Health/MensHealthNews/story?id = 7911505.

28. See, for example, "Mediterranean Diet Can Help Improve Sexual Health in Men," Health in 30 Website, accessed December 31, 2014, http://healthin30.com/2010/02/mediterranean-diet-can-help-improve-sexual-health-in-men/; Georgios Tsivgoulis et al., "Adherence to a Mediterranean Diet and Risk of Incident Cognitive Impairment," *Neurology* 80, no. 18 (2013): 1684–92.

29. Ancel and Margaret Keys, *Eat Well and Stay Well* (New York: Doubleday, 1959); *How to Eat Well and Stay Well the Mediterranean Way* (1975).

30. Todd Tucker, *The Great Starvation Experiment: Ancel Keys and the Men Who Starved for Science* (Minneapolis: University of Minnesota Press, 2006).

31. Frank Bruni, "Just How Good Can Italy Get?" *New York Times,* October 25, 2006, 1F, www.nytimes.com/2006/10/25/dining/25ital.html. Martha Rose Shulman, "Collard Greens: Rethinking a Southern Classic," *New York Times,* October 26, 2009, www.nytimes.com/2009/10/26/health/26recipehealth.html.

32. Laura Knowlton-Le Roux, "Reading American Fat in France: Obesity and Food Culture," *European Journal of American Studies* 2, no. 2 (2007).

33. Elaine Sciolino, "France Battles a Problem that Grows and Grows: Fat," *New York Times*, January 25, 2006, accessed December 31, 2014, www.nytimes.com/2006/01/25/international/europe/25obese.html; although a ban on vending machines in schools has helped level off child obesity rates, www.nytimes.com/2008/05/15/world/europe/15iht-health.4.12927785.html.

34. David Goodman, E. Melanie DuPuis, and Michael K. Goodman, *Alternative Food Networks: Knowledge, Practice and Politics* (New York: Routledge, 2012).

35. M. B. Marini and Patrick Mooney, "Rural Economies," in *Handbook of Rural Studies*, ed. Paul Cloke, Terry Marsden, and Patrick Mooney (London: Sage, 2006), 91–103.

36. Janet Chrzan, "Culinary Tourism in Tuscany: Media Fantasies, Imagined Traditions and Transformative Travel," in *Tourism and Museum: Sanitas per Aquas, Spas, Lifestyles and Foodways*, ed. Patricia Lysaght (Innsbruck: StudienVerlag, 2008), 236.

37. Graham Robb, *The Discovery of France: A Historical Geography* (New York: W. W. Norton, 2008).

38. Rachel Laudan, "Slow Food: The French Terroir Strategy, and Culinary Modernism—An Essay Review of Carlos Petrini, *Slow Food: The Case for Taste*, trans. William McCuaig," *Food Culture and Society: An International Journal of Multidisciplinary Research* 7, no. 2 (2004): 133–44.

39. Brahm Ahmadi, "Slow Food Needs Reality Check, Not Makeover," *Brahm's Blog*, July 28, 2008, accessed October 3, 2008, http://peoplesgrocery.org/brahm/peoples-grocery/slow-food-nyt.

40. Kim Severson, "Slow Food Savors Its Big Moment," *New York Times*, July 23, 2008, www.nytimes.com/2008/07/23/dining/23slow.html.

41. Frank Fitzpatrick, "Medal-worthy Food Slowing Down in Tasty Turin," *Philadelphia Inquirer* and *New York Times*, February 23, 2006.

42. Kim Severson, "For U.S. Food Elite, an Unlikely (Crowned) Hero," *New York Times*, April 25, 2007, 5; Patric Kuh, "Alice, Let's Eat," *New York Times*, June 3, 2007, 32; Fitzpatrick, "Medal-worthy Food."

43. Pollan, *Omnivore's Dilemma*.

CHAPTER 6: THE TROUBLE WITH PURITY

1. William Cronon, "The Trouble with Wilderness; or, Getting Back to the Wrong Nature," in *Uncommon Ground: Rethinking the Human Place in Nature*, ed. William Cronon (New York: W. W. Norton, 1995), 69.

2. "Our Mission" page on The Breakthrough website, accessed February 28, 2015, http://thebreakthrough.org/about/mission/.

3. Thomas Gieryn, "Boundary-Work and the Demarcation of Science from Non-Science: Strains and Interests in Professional Ideologies of Scientists," *American Sociological Review* 48 (1983): 781.

4. Michele Lamont and Virag Molnar, "The Study of Boundaries in the Social Sciences," *American Review of Sociology* 28 (2002): 168.

5. Pierre Bourdieu, *Distinction: A Social Critique of the Judgment of Taste* (New York: Routledge, 1984).

6. Martin Melosi, *The Sanitary City: Environmental Services in Urban America from Colonial Times to the Present* (Pittsburgh: University of Pittsburgh Press, 2008); Joel Tarr, *The Search for the Ultimate Sink: Urban Pollution in Historical Perspective* (Akron, OH: University of Akron Press, 1996).

7. Melosi, *Sanitary City;* Tarr, *Search for the Ultimate Sink.*

8. Marc Law and Gary D. Libecap, *The Determinants of Progressive Era Reform: The Pure Food and Drugs Act of 1906* (Chicago: University of Chicago Press, 2004).

9. Alejandro Junger, *Clean Gut: The Breakthrough Plan for Eliminating the Root Cause of Disease and Revolutionizing Your Health* (New York: Harcourt, 2013).

10. Ruben D. Acosta and Brooks D. Cash, "Clinical Effects of Colonic Cleansing for General Health Promotion: A Systematic Review," *American Journal of Gastroenterology* 104 (2009): 2835.

11. Dara Mohammadi, "You Can't Detox Your Body. It's a Myth. So How Do You Get Healthy?" *The Guardian,* December 5, 2014, accessed January 13, 2015, www.theguardian.com/lifeandstyle/2014/dec/05/detox-myth-health-diet-science-ignorance?CMP = soc_567.

12. Acosta and Cash, "Clinical Effects of Colonic Cleansing," 2835.

13. Bernard Dixon, "Detox: A Mass Delusion," *Lancet* 5, no. 5 (2005): 261.

14. Susan Bordo, *Unbearable Weight: Feminism, Western Culture and the Body* (Berkeley: University of California Press, 2004).

15. James C. Whorton, *Inner Hygiene: Constipation and the Pursuit of Health in Modern Society* (New York: Oxford University Press, 2000).

16. Tom Philpott, "Why Freakonomics Is Wrong about Cantaloupes," *Mother Jones,* accessed October 21, 2011, www.motherjones.com/tom-philpott/2011/10/freakonomics-cantaloupes-listeria.

17. Personal interview with Keith Schneider, April 22, 2015.

18. Ibid.

19. Steve Sexton, "Lessons of the *Listeria* Outbreak: Do Locavores Make Us Less Safe?" *Freakonomics Blog,* October 20, 2011, accessed November 23, 2014. http://freakonomics.com/2011/10/20/lessons-of-the-listeria-outbreak-do-locavores-make-us-less-safe/comment-page-5/.

20. 2011 cantaloupe acreage data in National Agricultural Statistics Service, Colorado Field Office, *Colorado Agricultural Statistics,* accessed January 14, 2015, www.nass.usda.gov/Statistics_by_State/Colorado/Publications/Annual_Statistical_Bulletin/Bulletin2014.pdf.

21. Susan A. Mann and James M. Dickinson, "Obstacles to the Development of a Capitalist Agriculture," *Journal of Peasant Studies* 5, no. 4 (1978).

22. "List of Selected Multistate Foodborne Outbreak Investigations," accessed January 15, 2014, www.cdc.gov/foodsafety/outbreaks/multistate-outbreaks

/outbreaks-list.html. As the list of total outbreaks shows, most are localized and due to handling, such as shared food at church socials, private parties, and company picnics, as well as restaurants. Multistate, large-scale foodborne outbreaks due to fresh produce are on this "selected" list.

23. Personal interview with Keith Schneider, April 22, 2015.

24. Jim Prevor, "Pundit's Mailbag: The End of the Yeoman Farmer? Does Society Care Enough about PTI and FSMA to Put the Small Farmer Out of Business?" July 22, 2013, accessed April 22, 2015, www.perishablepundit.com/index.php.

25. *Harvey v. Veneman*, 35 ELR 20022, no. 04–1379 (1st Cir., January 26, 2005).

26. Organic Foods Production Act of 1990, Title XXI of the Food, Agriculture, Conservation, and Trade Act of 1990 (Public Law 101–624, November 28, 1990).

27. Timothy Vos, "Visions of the Middle Landscape: Organic Farming and the Politics of Nature," *Agriculture and Human Values* 17, no. 3 (2000).

28. Michael Pollan, "Behind the Organic-Industrial Complex," *New York Times Magazine* section, May 13, 2001, accessed January 18, 2015, www.nytimes.com/2001/05/13/magazine/13ORGANIC.html.

29. Samuel Fromartz, *Organic, Inc.: Natural Foods and How They Grew* (Orlando: Harcourt, 2006).

30. *Harvey v. Veneman*.

31. Organic Trade Association, *USDA: Support Organic Agriculture and the Organic Industry through Targeted Programs: Comments of the Organic Trade Association on "Notice of Meetings and Request for Comments,"* 2005b, Federal Register, Friday, June 17, 2005, accessed January 15, 2008, www.ota.com/pp/otaposition/frc/USDA12–30–05.html.

32. USDA, Agricultural Marketing Service, National Organic Program, "Sunset Review and Renewal Process," accessed January 12, 2015, www.ams.usda.gov/AMSv1.0/getfile?dDocName=STELPRDC5107636.

33. I have discussed this case in two other publications, specifically E. Melanie DuPuis and Sean Gillon, "Alternative Modes of Governance: Organic as Civic Engagement," *Agriculture and Human Values* 26, nos. 1–2 (2009): 43–56; and David Goodman, E. Melanie DuPuis, and Michael K. Goodman, *Alternative Food Networks: Knowledge, Practice, and Politics* (New York: Routledge, 2012). See also, Thomas A. Lyson, *Civic Agriculture: Reconnecting Farm, Food, and Community* (Medford, MA: Tufts University Press, 2004).

34. James Riddle, "Open Letter to USDA: Struggle over Safeguarding Organic Standards Is Not Over," 2004, accessed January 15, 2015, www.organicconsumers.org/SOS/riddle060204.cfm.

35. US Department of Agriculture, National Organic Standards Board Hearings, Washington, DC, March 28, 2007, 349.

36. Coni Francis, "Comments at National Organic Standards Board Meeting," Public Hearing, March 28, 2007.

37. James Riddle, "Comments at National Organic Standards Board Meeting." Public Hearing, March 28, 2007.

38. Daniel Jaffee and Philip H. Howard, "Corporate Cooptation of Organic and Fair Trade Standards," *Agriculture and Human Values* 27, no. 4 (2010): 387–99.

39. www.progressivedairy.com/indes.php?option=com_contect&view=article&id=803:0607-pd-organic-dairy-industry-approaches-life-with-harveyq&catid=99:part-articles, accessed April 23, 2013.

40. Federal Register vol. 23, no. 207, October 24, 2008. Agricultural Marketing Service 7 CFR Part 205 National Organic Program (NOP)—Access to Pasture (Livestock) Proposed Rule.

41. Stephen R. Gliessman, *Agroecology: The Ecology of Sustainable Food Systems,* 2nd ed. (Boca Raton, FL: CRC Press, 2006), 384.

42. Survey responses cited in www.ams.usda.gov/AMSv1.0, accessed May 3, 2015.

43. David Goodman, E. Melanie DuPuis, and Michael K Goodman, *Alternative Food Networks: Knowledge, Practice, and Politics* (New York: Routledge, 2012), 169.

44. Albert O. Hirschman, *Exit, Voice, and Loyalty: Responses to Decline in Firms, Organizations, and States* (Boston: Harvard University Press, 1970).

45. "Horizon 'Organic' Factory Farm Accused of Improprieties, Again," *Cornucopia Institute,* February 14, 2014, accessed January 14, 2015, www.cornucopia.org/2014/02/horizon-organic-factory-farm-accused-improprieties/.

46. Roberta Sassatelli and Alan Scott, "Novel Food, New Markets and Trust Regimes: Responses to the Erosion of Consumers' Confidence in Austria, Italy and the UK," *European Societies* 3, no. 2 (2001); *St. Louis Post-Dispatch,* March 4, 2007, A1.

47. Patricia Allen, *Together at the Table: Sustainability and Sustenance in the American Agrifood System* (University Park: Penn State University Press, 2004).

CHAPTER 7: FERMENT: AN ECOLOGY OF THE BODY

1. Joshua Lederberg, "Infectious History," *Science* 288, no. 5464 (2000).

2. George Johnson, "Cancer's Secrets Come into Sharper Focus," *New York Times,* August 15, 2011, www.nytimes.com/2011/08/16/health/16cancer.html.

3. Donna Haraway, *The Companion Species Manifesto: Dogs, People, and Significant Otherness* (Chicago: Prickly Paradigm Press, 2003).

4. M. Hattori and T.D. Taylor, "The Human Intestinal Microbiome: A New Frontier of Human Biology," *DNA Research* 16, no. 1 (2009); J.I. Gordon et al., "Extending Our View of Self: The Human Gut Microbiome Initiative," 2005, www.genome.gov/10002154; P.B. Eckburg et al., "Diversity of the Human Intestinal Microbial Flora," *Science* 308 (2005): 1635–38; Lederberg, "Infectious History."

5. Elizabeth K. Costello, Keaton Stagaman, Les Dethlefsen, Brendan J.M. Bohannan, and David A. Relman, "The Application of Ecological Theory toward an Understanding of the Human Microbiome," *Science* 8 (June 2012): 336.

6. Elizabeth A. Grice and Julie A. Segre, "The Skin Microbiome," *Natural Reviews Microbiology* 9 (2011): 244.

7. Emily B. Hollister, Chunxu Gao, and James Versalovic, "Compositional and Functional Features of the Gastrointestinal Microbiome and Their Effects on Human Health," *Gastroenterology* 146, no. 6 (May 2014).

8. Julie Parsonnet, "Evolution of the Human Rain Forest: We Are What Eats Us," presentation to MIT Club of Northern California, January, 2012.

9. Ilseung Cho and Martin J. Blaser, "The Human Microbiome: At the Interface of Health and Disease," *Nature Reviews Genetics* 13, no. 4 (2012).

10. Lawrence A. David et al., "Diet Rapidly and Reproducibly Alters the Human Gut Microbiome," *Nature* 505 (January 23, 2014).

11. Sarah Haskin, "Target Women: Yogurt" video, accessed January 18, 2015, www.youtube.com/watch?v = Sf_roIC9Pso.

12. http://docsontheweb.blogspot.com/2008/04/dannon-activia-yogurt-and-bifidus.html, accessed September 10, 2008.

13. Emily Martin, "The Egg and the Sperm: How Science Has Constructed a Romance Based on Stereotypical Male-Female Roles," *Signs* 16, no. 3 (1991).

14. Aaron Bobrow-Strain, *White Bread: A Social History of the Store-bought Loaf* (Boston: Beacon, 2013).

15. Haraway, *Companion Species Manifesto.*

16. Aldo Leopold, "Thinking Like a Mountain," in *A Sand County Almanac* (New York: Random House, 1966), 140.

17. Ibid., 141.

18. While *A Sand County Almanac* was published in 1947, the essays were written over a long period. According to Susan Flader in her essay, "Thinking Like a Mountain: Aldo Leopold and the Evolution of an Ecological Attitude toward Deer, Wolves, and Forests," *Natural Resource Journal* (1974): 284, Leopold's "Thinking Like a Mountain" was first drafted in 1944.

19. Lijbert Brussaard, Peter C. de Ruiter, and George G. Brown, "Soil Biodiversity for Agricultural Sustainability," *Agriculture, Ecosystems and Environment* 121 (2007). 234.

20. Volker Mai and J. Glenn Morris, Jr., "Colonic Bacterial Flora: Changing Understandings in the Molecular Age," *Journal of Nutrition* 134, no. 2 (2004): 462.

21. Hattori and Taylor, "Human Intestinal Microbiome."

22. Erik Swyngedouw, "Apocalypse Forever? Post-political Populism and the Spectre of Climate Change," *Theory, Culture and Society* 27, nos. 2–3 (2010): 222; Julie Guthman, "Doing Justice to Bodies? Reflections on Food Justice, Race, and Biology," *Antipode* 46, no. 5 (2014): 1156.

23. Hans-Jörg Rheinberger, *Toward a History of Epistemic Things* (Stanford, CA: Stanford University Press, 1997); Dominique Laporte, *History of Shit* (Cambridge, MA: MIT Press, 2002).

24. M. Callon and J. Law, "Agency and the Hybrid 'Collectif'," *South Atlantic Quarterly* 94, no. 2 (1995).

25. Haraway, *Companion Species Manifesto.*

26. Joan Jacobs Brumberg, "The Appetite as Voice," in *Food and Culture: A Reader,* ed. Carole Counihan and Peggy Van Esterik (New York: Routledge, 1997).

27. Gary Gerstle, *American Crucible: Race and Nation in the Twentieth Century* (Princeton, NJ: Princeton University Press, 2001).

28. Juergen Habermas, *Communication and the Evolution of Society* (Boston: Beacon Press, 1979).

29. John S. Dryzek, *Deliberative Democracy and Beyond: Liberals, Critics, and Contestations* (New York: Oxford University Press, 2000).

30. Ulrich Beck et al., *Reflexive Modernization: Politics and Aesthetics in the Modern Social Order* (Stanford, CA: Stanford University Press, 1994).

31. Douglas S. Massey and Nancy A. Denton, *American Apartheid: Segregation and the Making of the Underclass* (Cambridge, MA: Harvard University Press, 1993).

32. Will Kymlicka, *Contemporary Political Philosophy: An Introduction* (New York: Oxford University Press, 2002), 259; see also Iris Marion Young, *Inclusion and Democracy* (New York: Oxford University Press, 2000).

33. Kymlicka, *Contemporary Political Philosophy*, 230.

34. Charles Taylor, "The Politics of Recognition," in *Multiculturalism: Examining the Politics of Recognition* (Princeton, NJ: Princeton University Press, 1994), 25.

35. Nancy Fraser, "From Redistribution to Recognition: Dilemmas of Justice in a 'Post-Socialist' Age," *New Left Review* 212 (1995); John Brown-Childs, *Transcommunality: From the Politics of Conversion to the Ethics of Respect* (Philadelphia: Temple University Press, 2003).

36. Brown-Childs, *Transcommunality*.

CHAPTER 8: TOWARD A FERMENTIVE POLITICS

1. Valerie A. Brown et al., *Tackling Wicked Problems: Through the Transdisciplinary Imagination* (New York: Routledge, 2010), 6.

2. Silvio O. Funtowicz and Jerome R. Ravetz, "Science for the Post-normal Age," *Futures* 25, no. 7 (1993): 750.

3. Ibid., 741.

4. Ibid., 751.

5. Bruno Latour, "From the World of Science to the World of Research," *Science* 10 280, no. 5361 (April 1988): 209.

6. For a more detailed discussion of this case, see David Goodman, E. Melanie DuPuis, and Michael K. Goodman, *Alternative Food Networks: Knowledge, Practice, and Politics* (New York: Routledge, 2012).

7. E. Melanie DuPuis, *Nature's Perfect Food: How Milk Became America's Drink* (New York: New York University Press, 2002).

8. Bruno Latour, "Visualization and Cognition: Drawing Things Together," *Knowledge and Society* 6 (1986).

9. Goodman et al., *Alternative Food Networks*, 193.

10. Francois Melard, Nathalie Semal, and Dorothee Denayer, "The Exploration of Environmental Controversies for Pedagogical Purposes: How to Learn Again to

Slow Down and Hesitate," May 20, 2014, Unité SEED—Département de sciences et gestion de l'environnement.

11. Many researchers of fair trade have made this point, including Laura Raynolds, Peter Taylor, Chris Bacon, and Mike Goodman.

12. Helga Nowotny, Peter Scott, and Michael Gibbons, *Re-thinking Science: Knowledge and the Public in an Age of Uncertainty* (Cambridge: Polity, 2001), 1.

13. Latour, "World of Science," 208.

BIBLIOGRAPHY

Abbott, Richard H. 1984. "A Yankee Views the Organization of the Republican Party in South Carolina, July 1867." *South Carolina Historical Society* 85, no. 3: 244–50.

———. 1991. *Cotton and Capital: Boston Businessmen and Antislavery Reform, 1854–1868.* Amherst: University of Massachusetts Press.

Acosta, Ruben D., and Brooks D. Cash. 2009. "Clinical Effects of Colonic Cleansing for General Health Promotion: A Systematic Review." *American Journal of Gastroenterology* 104: 2835.

Adams, John. 1774. *Novanglus Letters, No. III.*

Ahn A. C., M. Tewari, C. S. Poon, and R. S. Phillips. 2006. "The Limits of Reductionism in Medicine: Could Systems Biology Offer an Alternative?" *PLoS Med* 3, no. 6: e208.

Alcott, Louisa May. 1981. *Transcendental Wild Oats and Excerpts from the Fruitlands Diary.* Harvard, MA: Harvard Common Press.

Allen, Patricia. 2004. *Together at the Table: Sustainability and Sustenance in the American Agrifood System.* University Park: Penn State University Press.

Almaguer, Tomás. 2008. *Racial Fault Lines: The Historical Origins of White Supremacy in California.* Berkeley: University of California Press.

Anderson, Eugene N. 1988. *The Food of China.* New Haven, CT: Yale University Press.

Anon. 1869. "The Non-Beef-Eating Nations." *Saturday Evening Post,* November 13, 8.

Appadurai, Arjun. 1981. "Gastropolitics in Hindu South Asia." *American Ethnologist* 8: 494–511.

Arikha, Noga. 2007. *Passions and Tempers: A History of the Humours.* New York: Ecco.

Arnold, David. 2010. "British India and the 'Beriberi Problem,' 1798–1942." *Medical History* 54, no. 3: 295–314.

Atwater, W. O. 1888. "A Pecuniary Economy of Food: The Chemistry of Food and Nutrition." *The Century: A Popular Quarterly* 35, no. 3: 437–46.

———. 1888. "What We Should Eat." *The Century: A Popular Quarterly* 36: 257–64.

Barfoot, Chas. H. 2014. *Aimee Semple McPherson and the Making of Modern Pentecostalism, 1890–1926.* New York: Routledge.

Baudrillard, Jean. 1988. *America.* New York: Verso.

Beck, Ulrich, et al. 1994. *Reflexive Modernization: Politics and Aesthetics in the Modern Social Order.* Stanford, CA: Stanford University Press.

Beecher, Catharine, and Harriet Beecher Stowe. 2008. *The American Woman's Home: Principles of Domestic Science.* Carlisle, MA: Applewood Books.

Berry, Wendell. 2009. "The Pleasures of Eating." In *Bringing It to the Table: On Farming and Food.* Berkeley: Counterpoint Press.

Biltekoff, Charlotte. 2013. *Eating Right in America: The Cultural Politics of Food and Health.* Durham, NC: Duke University Press Books.

Bloem, Jaap, Ton Schouten, Wim Didden, Gerard Jagers op Akkerhuis, Harm Keidel, Michiel Rutgers, and Ton Breure. 2003. "Measuring Soil Biodiversity: Experiences, Impediments and Research Needs." OECD Expert Meeting on Soil Erosion and Soil Biodiversity Indicators, March 25–28, Rome, Italy.

Bobrow-Strain, Aaron. 2013. *White Bread: A Social History of the Store-Bought Loaf.* Boston: Beacon Press.

Bordo, Susan. 2004. *Unbearable Weight: Feminism, Western Culture and the Body.* Berkeley: University of California Press.

Bourdieu, Pierre. 1984. *Distinction: A Social Critique of the Judgement of Taste.* New York: Routledge.

Brabec, Elizabeth, and Sharon Richardson. 2007. "A Clash of Cultures: The Landscape of the Sea Island Gullah." *Landscape Journal* 26: 1–7.

Brantley, Cynthia. 1997. "Kikiyu-Maasai Nutrition and Colonial Science: The Orr and Gilks Study in the Late 1920s Revisited." *International Journal of African Historical Studies* 30: 49–86.

———. 2002. *Feeding Families: African Realities and British Ideas of Nutrition and Development in Early Colonial Africa.* Portsmouth, NH: Heinemann.

Brewer, Priscilla J. 1984. "The Demographic Features of the Shaker Decline, 1787–1900." *Journal of Interdisciplinary History* 15: 31–52.

Brodsky, Alyn. 2004. *Benjamin Rush: Patriot and Physician.* New York: Truman Talley.

Brown, Valerie A., John A. Harris, and Jacqueline Y. Russell. 2010. *Tackling Wicked Problems: Through the Transdisciplinary Imagination.* Washington, DC: Earthscan.

Brown-Childs, John. 2003. *Transcommunality: From the Politics of Conversion.* Philadelphia: Temple University Press.

Brumberg, Joan Jacobs. 1997. "The Appetite as Voice." In *Food and Culture: A Reader,* edited by Carole Counihan and Peggy Van Esterik. New York: Routledge.

Bruni, Frank. 2006. "Just How Good Can Italy Get?" *New York Times,* October 25, 1F.

Brussaard, Lijbert, Peter C. de Ruiter, and George G. Brown. 2007. "Soil Biodiversity for Agricultural Sustainability." *Agriculture, Ecosystems and Environment* 121: 233–44.

Buck, John L. 1930. *Chinese Farm Economy.* Chicago: University of Chicago Press.

Bushman, Richard Lyman. 2005. *Joseph Smith: Rough Stone Rolling.* New York: Alfred A. Knopf.

Butterfield, L. H. 1951. *Letters of Benjamin Rush.* Princeton, NJ: Princeton University Press.

Callon, Michel, and John Law. 1995. "Agency and the Hybrid 'Collectif.'" *South Atlantic Quarterly* 94, no. 2: 481–507.

Chen, Thomas S. N., and Peter S. Y. Chen. 1989. "Intestinal Autointoxication: A Medical Leitmotif." *Journal of Clinical Gastroenterology* 11, no. 4: 367–488.

Chesnut, Mary Boykin. 1984. *The Private Mary Chesnut: The Unpublished Civil War Diaries.* New York: Oxford University Press.

Cho, Ilseung, and Martin J. Blaser. 2012. "The Human Microbiome: At the Interface of Health and Disease." *Nature Reviews Genetics* 13, no. 4: 260–70.

Chrzan, Janet. 2008. "Culinary Tourism in Tuscany: Media Fantasies, Imagined Traditions and Transformative Travel." In *Tourism and Museum: Sanitas per Aquas, Spas, Lifestyles and Foodways,* edited by Patricia Lysaght, 235–51. Innsbruck: StudienVerlag.

Claybaugh, Amanda. 2006. "Toward a New Transatlanticism: Dickens in the United States." *Victorian Studies* 8, no. 3: 439–60.

Clement, Priscilla Ferguson. 1997. *Growing Pains: Children in the Industrial Age, 1850–1890.* New York: Twayne.

Cohen, Lizabeth. 2003. *A Consumers' Republic: The Politics of Mass Consumption in Postwar America.* New York: Knopf.

Colt, George Howe. 2003. *The Big House: A Century in the Life of an American Summer Home.* New York: Scribner.

Coppin, Clayton A., and Jack C. High. 1999. *The Politics of Purity: Harvey Washington Wiley and the Origins of Federal Food Policy.* Ann Arbor: University of Michigan Press.

Corbin, Alain. 1986. *The Foul and the Fragrant: Odor and the French Social Imagination.* Cambridge, MA: Harvard University Press.

Corson, Juliet. 1883. *Cooking School Text Book; and Housekeepers' Guide to Cookery and Kitchen Management.* New York: O. Judd.

Costello, Elizabeth K., Keaton Stagaman, Les Dethlefsen, Brendan J. M. Bohannan, and David A. Relman. 2012. "The Application of Ecological Theory toward an Understanding of the Human Microbiome." *Science* 336, no. 6086: 1255–62.

Cotler, Amy. 2009. *The Locavore Way: Discover and Enjoy the Pleasures of Locally Grown Food.* North Adams, MA: Storey.

Coveney, John. 2000. *Food, Morals and Meaning: The Pleasures and Anxiety of Eating.* New York: Routledge.

Covey, Herbert C., and Dwight Eisnach. 2009. *What the Slaves Ate: Recollections of African American Foods and Foodways from the Slave Narratives.* Santa Barbara, CA: ABC-CLIO.

Cronon, William. 1995. "The Trouble with Wilderness; or, Getting Back to the Wrong Nature." In *Uncommon Ground: Rethinking the Human Place in Nature,* edited by William Cronon, 69–90. New York: W. W. Norton.

Cross, Whitney. 1981. *The Burned-Over District: The Social and Intellectual History of Enthusiastic Religion in Western New York, 1800–1850.* New York: Octagon.

Currell, Susan, and Christina Cogdell. 2006. *Popular Eugenics: National Efficiency and American Mass Culture in the 1930s.* Athens: Ohio University Press.

Dalgaard, Tommy, Nicholas J. Hutchings, and John R. Porter. 2003. "Agroecology, Scaling and Interdisciplinarity." *Agriculture, Ecosystems and Environment* 100: 39–51.

Danone Institute. N.d. "Historical Commitment of the Danone Institute to Health." Accessed September 10, 2008. www.danoneinstitute.org/about_danone_institute/history.php.

David, Lawrence A., et al. 2014. "Diet Rapidly and Reproducibly Alters the Human Gut Microbiome." *Nature* 505: 559–63.

Davis, David Brion. 1999. *The Problem of Slavery in the Age of Revolution.* New York: Oxford University Press.

Davis, Mike. 2002. *Late Victorian Holocausts: El Niño Famines and the Making of the Third World.* New York: Verso.

Day, Aidan. 2012. *Romanticism: The New Critical Idiom.* London, New York: Routledge Taylor & Francis Group.

Day, Harry G. and Harry J. Prebluda. 1980. "E. V. McCollum: 'Lamplighter' in Public and Professional Understanding of Nutrition." *Agricultural History* 54, no. 1: 149–56.

Debs, Eugene V. 1990. *Letters of Eugene V. Debs,* vol. 1. Edited by J. Robert Constantine. Champaign: University of Illinois Press.

D'Elia, Donald J. 1974. "Benjamin Rush: Philosopher of the American Revolution." *Transactions of the American Philosophical Society* 64, no. 5.

Dimand, Robert W. 1997. "Irving Fisher and Modern Macroeconomics." *American Economic Review* 87, no. 2: 442–44.

Dimand, Robert W. and John Geanakoplos. 2005. "Celebrating Irving Fisher: The Legacy of a Great Economist." *American Journal of Economics and Sociology* 64, no. 1: 3–18.

Diner, Hasia R. 2001. *Hungering for America: Italian, Irish, and Jewish Foodways in the Age of Migration.* Cambridge, MA: Harvard University Press.

Dixon, Bernard. 2005. "Detox: A Mass Delusion." *Lancet* 5, no. 5: 261.

Douglas, Mary. 1996. *Purity and Danger: An Analysis of Concepts of Pollution and Taboo.* New York: Praeger.

Dryzek, John S. 2000. *Deliberative Democracy and Beyond: Liberals, Critics, and Contestations.* New York: Oxford University Press.

DuPuis, E. Melanie. 2002. *Nature's Perfect Food: How Milk Became America's Drink.* New York: New York University Press.

———. 2007. "Angels and Vegetables: A Brief History of Food Advice in America." *Gastronomica: The Journal of Critical Food Studies* 7, no. 3: 34–44.

——— and Sean Gillon. 2009. "Alternative Modes of Governance: Organic as Civic Engagement." *Agriculture and Human Values* 26, nos. 1–2: 43–56.

Eckburg, P. B., E. M. Bik, C. N. Bernstein, E. Purdom, L. Dethlefsen, M. Sargent, S. R. Gill, K. E. Nelson, and D. A. Relman. 2005. "Diversity of the Human Intestinal Microbial Flora." *Science* 308: 1635–38.

Edwards, Richards. 1980. *Contested Terrain.* New York: Basic Books.

Egan, Kristen R. 2011. "Conservation and Cleanliness: Racial and Environmental Purity in Ellen Richards and Charlotte Perkins Gilman." *WSQ: Women's Studies Quarterly* 39, no. 3: 77–92.

Ehart, Bob. 2013. "As FDA Implements FSMA, NASDA Seeks Support to Get the Rules Right." *Food Safety News,* September 24. www.foodsafetynews.com/2013/09/as-fda-implements-fsma-nasda-seeks-support-to-get-the-rules-right/#.VC67_SldWEy.

Emerson, Ralph Waldo. 1887. *New England Reformers and Divinity College Address.* New York: John B. Alden.

Farina, John, ed. 1988. *Isaac T. Hecker, The Diary: Romantic Religion in Ante-bellum America.* New York: Paulist Press.

Faust, Drew Gilpin. 1979. "A Southern Stewardship: The Intellectual and the Pro-slavery Argument." *American Quarterly* 31, no. 1: 63–80.

Finney, Carolyn. 2014. *Black Faces, White Spaces: Reimagining the Relationship of African Americans to the Great Outdoors.* Chapel Hill: University of North Carolina Press.

Fitzpatrick, Frank. 2006. "Medal-worthy Food: Slowing Down in Tasty Turin." *Philly.com,* February 23.

Flynn, Dan. 2013. "State Ag Directors Want Congress to Give FDA More Time on FSMA Rules." *Food Safety News,* September 25. www.foodsafetynews.com/2013/09/state-ag-directors-want-congress-to-give-fda-more-time/#.VC67BCldWEy.

Foner, Eric. 1980. *Politics and Ideology in the Age of the Civil War.* New York: Oxford University Press.

———. 1995. *Free Soil, Free Labor, Free Men: The Ideology of the Republican Party Before the Civil War.* New York: Oxford University Press.

——— and Olivia Mahoney. 1997. *America's Reconstruction: People and Politics after the Civil War.* Baton Rouge: LSU Press.

Fraser, Nancy. 1995. "From Redistribution to Recognition: Dilemmas of Justice in a 'Post-Socialist' Age." *New Left Review* 212: 68–93.

Fromartz, Samuel. 2006. *Organic, Inc.: Natural Foods and How They Grew.* Orlando: Harcourt.

Funtowicz, Silvio O., and Jerome R. Ravetz. 1993. "Science for the Post-normal Age." *Futures* 25, no. 7: 739–824.

Furstenberg, Francois. 2003. "Beyond Freedom and Slavery: Autonomy, Virtue, and Resistance in Early American Political Discourse." *Journal of American History* 89, no. 4: 1295–1330.

Galton, Francis. 1883. *Inquiries into Human Faculty and Its Development.* New York: Macmillan.

Garrison, William Lloyd. 1861. "The War—Its Cause and Its Cure." *Liberator,* May 3.

Garvey, T. Gregory. 2006. *Creating the Culture of Reform in Antebellum America.* Athens: University of Georgia Press.

Gaytán, Marie Sarita. 2004. "Slow Food and New Local Imaginaries." *Food, Culture and Society: An International Journal of Multidisciplinary Research* 7, no. 2: 97–116.

Genovese, Elizabeth Fox. 1988. *Within the Plantation Household: Black and White Women of the Old South.* Chapel Hill: University of North Carolina Press.

Gerstle, Gary. 2001. *American Crucible: Race and Nation in the Twentieth Century.* Princeton, NJ: Princeton University Press.

Gieryn, Thomas. 1983. "Boundary-Work and the Demarcation of Science: Strains and Interests in the Professional Ideologies of Scientists." *American Sociological Review* 48: 781–95.

Gifford, K. Dun. 2002. "Dietary Fats, Eating Guides, and Public Policy: History, Critique, and Recommendations." *American Journal of Medicine* 113, no. 9: 89–106.

Gittell, Marilyn, and Teresa Shtob. 1980. "Changing Women's Roles in Political Volunteerism and Reform of the City," *Signs* 5, no. 3: S67–S78.

Gliessman, Stephen R. 2006. *Agroecology: The Ecology of Sustainable Food Systems,* 2nd ed. Boca Raton, FL: CRC Press.

Gompers, Samuel, and Herman Gutstadt. 1901. *Meat vs. Rice; American Manhhood against Asiatic Coolieism—Which Shall Survive?* San Francisco: American Federation of Labor.

Goodman, David, E. Melanie DuPuis, and Michael K. Goodman. 2012. *Alternative Food Networks: Knowledge, Practice, and Politics.* New York: Routledge.

Gordon, J. I., R. E. Ley, R. Wilson, E. Mardis, J. Xu, C. M. Fraser, and D. A. Relman. 2005. "Extending Our View of Self: The Human Gut Microbiome Initiative" (HGMI). www.genome.gov/10002154.

Graham, Sylvester. *Lectures on the Science of Human Life.* 1849. London: Boston, Marsh, Capen, Lyon & Webb.

Greenblatt, Steven Jay. 1980. *Renaissance Self-Fashioning: From More to Shakespeare.* Chicago: University of Chicago Press.

Grice, Elizabeth A., and Julia A. Segre. 2011. "The Skin Microbiome." *Natural Reviews Microbiology* 9: 244–53.

Gusfield, Joseph R. 1986. *Symbolic Crusade: Status Politics and the American Temperance Movement.* Urbana: University of Illinois Press.

Guthman, Julie. 2008. "Bringing Good Food to Others: Investigating the Subjects of Alternative Food Practice." *Cultural Geographies* 15, no. 4: 431–47.

———. 2014. "Doing Justice to Bodies? Reflections on Food Justice, Race, and Biology." *Antipode* 46, no. 5: 1153–71.

Guthman, Julie and E. Melanie DuPuis. 2006. "Embodying Neoliberalism: Economy, Culture, and the Politics of Fat." *Environment and Planning D: Society and Space* 24, no. 3: 427–48.

Gutman, Herbert G. 1973. "Work, Culture and Society in Industrializing America." *American Historical Review,* 531–87.

Habermas, Juergen. 1979. *Communication and the Evolution of Society.* Boston: Beacon Press.

Haraway, Donna. 2003. *The Companion Species Manifesto: Dogs, People, and Significant Otherness.* Chicago: Prickly Paradigm Press.

Harding, T. Swann. 1928. "Diet and Disease." *Scientific Monthly* 26, no. 2: 150–57.

Hartley, Isaac Smithson. 1976. *Memorial of Robert Milham Hartley.* New York: Arno Press.

Hattori, Masahira, and T. D. Taylor. 2009. "The Human Intestinal Microbiome: A New Frontier of Human Biology." *DNA Research* 16, no. 1: 1–12.

Hedrick, Ulysses P. 1933. *History of Agriculture in the State of New York.* Albany: New York State Agriculture Society.

Hendrickson, M., and W. D. Heffernan. 2002. "Opening Spaces through Relocalization: Locating Potential Resistance in the Weaknesses of the Global Food System." *Sociologia Ruralis* 42, no. 4: 347–69.

Hilliard, Sam Bowers. 1972. *Hog Meat and Hoecake: Food Supply in the Old South 1840–1860.* Carbondale: Southern Illinois University Press.

Hirschman, Albert O. 1970. *Exit, Voice, and Loyalty: Responses to Decline in Firms, Organizations, and States.* Boston: Harvard University Press.

Hoffman, Edwin D. 1956. "From Slavery to Self-Reliance: The Record of Achievement of the Freedmen of the Sea Island Region." *Journal of Negro History* 41: 8–42.

Hofstadter, Richard. 1963. *The Progressive Movement, 1900–1915.* Upper Saddle River, NJ: Prentice-Hall.

———. 1967. *The American Political Tradition and the Men Who Made It.* New York: Random House.

Hollister, Emily B., Chunxu Gao, and James Versalovic. 2014. "Compositional and Functional Features of the Gastrointestinal Microbiome and Their Effects on Human Health." *Gastroenterology* 146, no. 6: 1449–58.

Holt, D. B. 1998. "Does Cultural Capital Structure US Consumption?" *Journal of Consumer Research* 25, no. 1: 1–25.

Hopkins, Jim. 2003. "'Slow Food' Movement Gathers Momentum." *USA Today,* November 26, 1B.

"Horizon 'Organic' Factory Farm Accused of Improprieties, Again." 2014. *Cornucopia Institute,* February 14. www.cornucopia.org/2014/02/horizon-organic-factory-farm-accused-improprieties/.

Horowitz, Roger. 2006. *Putting Meat on the American Table.* Baltimore: JHU Press.

Hunt, Caroline Louisa. 1912. *The Life of Ellen H. Richards.* Boston: Whitcomb & Barrows.

Hunt, Lynn. 2008. *Inventing Human Rights: A History.* New York: W. W. Norton.

Hurston, Zora Neale. 1999. *Their Eyes Were Watching God.* New York: HarperCollins.

Jaffee, Daniel, and Philip H. Howard. 2010. "Corporate Cooptation of Organic and Fair Trade Standards." *Agriculture and Human Values* 27, no. 4: 387–99.

Johnson, George. 2011. "Cancer's Secrets Come into Sharper Focus." *New York Times,* August 16. www.nytimes.com/2011/08/16/health/16cancer.html.

Johnson, Paul E. 1978. *A Shopkeeper's Millennium: Society and Revivals in Rochester, NY, 1815–1837.* New York: Hill and Wang.

Junger, Alejandro. 2013. *Clean Gut: The Breakthrough Plan for Eliminating the Root Cause of Disease and Revolutionizing Your Health.* New York: Harcourt.

Kant, Ashima K., and Barry I. Graubard. 2004. "Eating Out in America, 1987–2000: Trends and Nutritional Correlates." *Preventive Medicine* 38, no. 2: 243–49.

Katz, Michael B., Michael K. Doucet, and Mark Stern. 1982. *The Social Organization of Early Capitalism*. Cambridge, MA: Harvard University Press.

Kaufman, Frederick. 2008. *A Short History of the American Stomach*. Orlando: Houghton Mifflin Harcourt.

Keys, Ancel. 1975. *How to Eat Well and Stay Well the Mediterranean Way*. Garden City, NJ: Doubleday.

Keys, Ancel, and Margaret Keys. 1959. *Eat Well and Stay Well*. Garden City, NJ: Doubleday.

King, Miriam, and Steven Ruggles. 1990. "American Immigration, Fertility, and Race Suicide at the Turn of the Century." *Journal of Interdisciplinary History* 20, no. 3: 347–69.

Kingsolver, Barbara, Camille Kingsolver, and Steven L. Hopp. 2008. *Animal, Vegetable, Miracle: A Year of Food Life*. New York: Harper Perennial.

Klein, Rachel N. 2001. "Harriet Beecher Stowe and the Domestication of Free Labor Ideology." *Legacy* 18, no. 2: 137–42.

Kloppenburg, Jack, John Hendrickson, and G. W. Stevenson. 1996. "Coming into the Foodshed." *Agriculture and Human Values* 13, no. 3: 33–42.

Knowlton-Le Roux, Laura. 2007. "Reading American Fat in France: Obesity and Food Culture." *European Journal of American Studies* 2, no. 2: 2–10.

Kuh, Patric. 2007. "Alice, Let's Eat." *New York Times,* June 3, 32.

Kymlicka, Will. 2002. *Contemporary Political Philosophy: An Introduction*. New York: Oxford University Press.

Lamont, Michele, and Annette Lareau. 1988. "Cultural Capital: Allusions, Gaps and Glissandos in Recent Theoretical Developments." *Sociological Theory* 6, no. 2: 153–68.

Lamont, Michele, and Virag Molnar. 2002. "The Study of Boundaries in the Social Sciences." *American Review of Sociology* 28: 167–95.

Lane, Charles, and Bronson Alcott. 1843. "The Consociate Family Life." *Liberator* 13: 152.

Lang, Tim, and Michael Heasman. 2004. *Food Wars: The Global Battle for Mouths Minds and Markets*. London: Earthscan.

Laporte, Dominique. 2002. *History of Shit*. Cambridge, MA: MIT Press.

Larson, Edward J. 1996. *Sex, Race, and Science: Eugenics in the Deep South*. Baltimore: Johns Hopkins University Press.

Latour, Bruno. 1986. "Visualization and Cognition: Drawing Things Together." *Knowledge and Society* 6: 1–40.

———. 1988. "From the World of Science to the World of Research." *Science* 10, no. 5361 (April): 208–9.

———. 1988. *The Pasteurization of France*. Cambridge, MA: Harvard University Press.

Laudan, Rachel. 2011. "Slow Food: The French Terroir Strategy, and Culinary Modernism—An Essay Review of Carlos Petrini, *Slow Food: The Case for Taste*, translated by William McCuaig." *Food Culture and Society: An International Journal of Multidisciplinary Research* 7, no. 2: 133–44.

Law, Marc, and Gary D. Libecap. 2004. *The Determinants of Progressive Era Reform: The Pure Food and Drugs Act of 1906*. Chicago: University of Chicago Press.

Lawrence, David A., et al. 2014. "Diet Rapidly and Reproducibly Alters the Human Gut Microbiome." *Nature 505* (January 23): 559–63.

League of Nations Mixed Committee on Nutrition. 1937. *Nutrition: Final Report of the Mixed Committee of the League of Nations on the Relation of Nutrition to Health, Agriculture, and Economic Policy*. Geneva.

Lederberg, Joshua. 2000. "Infectious History." *Science* 288, no. 5464: 287–93.

Leonard, Thomas C. 1986. *Power of the Press: The Birth of American Political Reporting*. Cary, NC: Oxford University Press.

———. 2005. "Retrospectives: Eugenics and Economics in the Progressive Era." *Journal of Economic Perspectives* 19, no. 4: 207–24.

Leopold, Aldo. 1966. "Thinking Like a Mountain." In *A Sand County Almanac*. New York: Random House.

Levenstein, Harvey. 1994. *A Paradox of Plenty: A Social History of Eating in Modern America*. Berkeley: University of California Press.

———. 2003. *Revolution at the Table: The Transformation of the American Diet*. Berkeley: University of California Press.

Levine, Lawrence W. 1988. *Highbrow / Lowbrow: The Emergence of Cultural Hierarchy in America*. Cambridge, MA: Harvard University Press.

Lipsitz, George. 2006. *The Possessive Investment in Whiteness*. Philadelphia: Temple University Press.

Lyson, Thomas A. 2004. *Civic Agriculture: Reconnecting Farm, Food, and Community*. Medford, MA: Tufts University Press.

MacArthur, Judith N. 1989. "Demon Rum on the Boards: Temperance Melodrama and the Tradition of Antebellum Reform." *Journal of the Early Republic* 9: 517–40.

Madison, James. 1788. *Federalist Papers, #51*.

Mai, Volker, and J. Glenn Morris, Jr. 2004. "Colonic Bacterial Flora: Changing Understandings in the Molecular Age." *Journal of Nutrition* 134, no. 2: 459–64.

Mann, Susan A., and James M. Dickinson. 1978. "Obstacles to the Development of a Capitalist Agriculture." *Journal of Peasant Studies* 5, no. 4: 466–81.

Marini, Matteo B., and Patrick Mooney. 2006. "Rural Economies." In *Handbook of Rural Studies*, edited by Paul Cloke, Terry Marsden, and Patrick Mooney. London: Sage.

Martin, Emily. 1991. "The Egg and the Sperm: How Science Has Constructed a Romance Based on Stereotypical Male-Female Roles." *Signs* 16, no. 3: 485–501.

Massey, Douglas S., and Nancy A. Denton. 1993. *American Apartheid: Segregation and the Making of the Underclass*. Cambridge, MA: Harvard University Press.

McArthur, Judith N. 1989. "Demon Rum on the Boards: Temperance Melodrama and the Tradition of Antebellum Reform." *Journal of the Early Republic* 9, no. 4 (Winter): 517–40.

McCann, Charles. 2012. *Order and Control in American Socio-Economic Thought: Social Scientists and Progressive-Era Reform.* New York: Routledge.

McCollum, Elmer Verner. 1919. *The Newer Knowledge of Nutrition: The Use of Food for the Preservation of Vitality and Health.* New York: McMillan.

McElroy, James L. 1977. "Social Control and Romantic Reform in Antebellum America: The Case of Rochester, New York." *New York History* 58: 17–46.

McEvedy, Allegra. 2007. "Organic Foods First Lady." *The Guardian* (London), May 2, 18. www.theguardian.com/environment/2007/may/02/food.foodanddrink.

McKelvey, Blake. 1971. "Flour Milling at Rochester." *Rochester History* 33: 10–34.

Mélard, Francois, Nathalie Semal, and Dorothee Denayer. 2014. *The Exploration of Environmental Controversies for Educational Purposes: How to Learn Again to Slow Down and Hesitate.* International Interdisciplinary Conference, "Teaching Complexity and Uncertainty on Environmental Issues-Practices, Theories and Products," Arlon, Belgium. http://orbi. ulg. ac. be/handle/2268/169671.

Melosi, Martin. 2008. *The Sanitary City: Environmental Services in Urban America from Colonial Times to the Present.* Pittsburgh: University of Pittsburgh Press.

Mohammadi, Dara. 2014. "You Can't Detox Your Body. It's a Myth. So How Do You Get Healthy?" *The Guardian,* December 5. www.theguardian.com /lifeandstyle/2014/dec/05/detox-myth-health-diet-science-ignorance?CMP = soc_ 567.

Mokdad, A. H., et al. 2001. "Prevalence of Obesity, Diabetes, and Obesity-related Health Risk Factors." *Journal of the American Medical Association* 289, no. 1: 76–79.

Molina, Natalia. 2006. *Fit to Be Citizens?: Public Health and Race in Los Angeles, 1879–1939.* Berkeley: University of California Press.

Moreira, Tiago, and Paolo Palladino. 2005. "Between Truth and Hope: On Parkinson's Disease, Neurotransplantation and the Production of the 'Self'." *History of the Human Sciences* 18, no. 3: 55–82.

Morgan, Edmund S. 1972. "Slavery and Freedom: The American Paradox." *Journal of American History* 59, no. 1: 5–29.

Morley, David, and Kuan-Hsing Chen. 1996. *Stuart Hall: Critical Dialogues in Cultural Studies.* New York: Routledge.

Morton, Timothy. 2006. "Joseph Ritson, Percy Shelley and the Making of Romantic Vegetarianism." *Romanticism* 12, no. 1: 56–61.

Mote, Frederick W. 1977. "Yuan and Ming." In *Food in Chinese Culture: Anthropological and Historical Perspectives,* edited by K. C. Chang, 193–257. New Haven, CT: Yale University Press.

Neely, Michelle C. 2013. "Embodied Politics: Antebellum Vegetarianism and the Dietary Economy of Walden." *American Literature* 85, no. 1: 33–60.

Nowotny, Helga, Peter Scott, and Michael Gibbons. 2001. *Re-thinking Science: Knowledge and the Public in an Age of Uncertainty.* Cambridge: Polity.

Numbers, Ronald L. 1992. *Prophetess of Health: Ellen G. White and the Origins of Seventh-Day Adventist Health Reform.* Knoxville: University of Tennessee Press.

O'Brien, Gerald V. 2003. "Indigestible Foods, Conquering Hordes and Waste Materials: Metaphors of Immigrants and the Early Immigration Restriction Debate in the United States." *Metaphor and Symbol* 18: 36–37.

Ogle, Maureen. 2013. *In Meat We Trust: An Unexpected History of Carnivore America.* Boston: Houghton Mifflin.

Pace, Joel. 2008. "Towards a Taxonomy of Transatlantic Romanticism(s)." *Literature Compass* 5, no. 2: 228–91.

Parsonnet, Julia. 2012. "Evolution of the Human Rain Forest: We are What Eats Us." Presentation to MIT Club of Northern California.

Pease, Jane H., and William H. Pease. 1972. "Confrontation and Abolition in the 1850s." *Journal of American History* 58, no. 4: 923–24.

Pegram, Thomas R. 1998. *Battling Demon Rum: The Struggle for a Dry America, 1800–1933.* Chicago: Ivan R. Dee.

Pendergrast, Mark. 2010. *Uncommon Grounds: The History of Coffee and How It Transformed Our World.* New York: Basic Books.

Pernick, Martin S. 1997. "Eugenics and Public Health in American History." *American Journal of Public Health* 87, no. 11: 1767–72.

Pessen, Edward. 1980. "How Different from Each Other Were the Antebellum North and South?" *American Historical Review* 85: 1119–49.

Petrini, Carlo. 2001. *Slow Food: A Case for Taste.* New York: Columbia University Press.

Philpott, Tom. 2011. "Why Freakonomics Is Wrong About Cantaloupes." *Mother Jones,* October 21. www.motherjones.com/tom-philpott/2011/10/freakonomics-cantaloupes-listeria.

Pickering, Andrew. 1993. "The Mangle of Practice: Agency and Emergence in the Sociology of Science." *American Journal of Sociology* 99, no. 3: 559–89.

Pietrykowski, Bruce. 2004. "You Are What You Eat: The Social Economy of the Slow Food Movement." *Review of Social Economy* 57, no. 3. www.informaworld.com/smpp/title~content = t713708792.

Pollan, Michael. 2006. *The Omnivore's Dilemma: A Natural History of Four Meals.* New York: Penguin.

Pollard, Sidney. 1963. "Factory Discipline in the Industrial Revolution." *Economic History Review* 16, no. 2: 254–71.

Polletta, Francesca. 2006. *It Was Like a Fever: Storytelling in Protest and Politics.* Chicago: University of Chicago Press.

Popkin, Barry M. 2001. "The Nutrition Transition and Obesity in the Developing World." *American Society for Nutritional Sciences* 131, no. 3.

Popkin, Barry M., and Colleen M. Doak. 1998. "The Obesity Epidemic Is a Worldwide Phenomenon." *Nutrition Reviews* 56, no. 4: 106–14.

Powell, Lawrence. 1980. *New Masters: Northern Planters during the Civil War and Reconstruction.* New Haven, CT: Yale University Press.

Randolph, Mary. 1836. *The Virginia Housewife, or Methodical Cook*. Baltimore: J. Plaskitt.

Reynolds, David S. 2008. *Waking Giant: America in the Age of Jackson*. New York: Harper Perennial.

Rheinberger, Hans-Jörg. 1997. *Toward a History of Epistemic Things*. Stanford, CA: Stanford University Press.

Richards, Ellen Swallow. 1910. *Euthenics, The Science of Controllable Environment: A Plea for Better Living Conditions as a First Step Toward Higher Human Efficiency*. Boston: Whitcomb & Barrows.

Ring, Natalie J. 2012. *The Problem South: Region, Empire and the New Liberal State, 1880–1930*. Athens: University of Georgia Press.

Robb, Graham. 2008. *The Discovery of France: A Historical Geography*. New York: W. W. Norton.

Rondon, M. R., R. M. Goodman, and J. Handelsman. 1999. "The Earth's Bounty: Assessing and Accessing Soil Microbial Diversity." *Trends in Biotechnology* 17, no. 10: 403–9.

Roy, Parama. 2002. "Meat-Eating, Masculinity, and Renunciation in India: A Gandhian Grammar of Diet." *Gender and History* 14, no. 1: 62–91.

Runes, Dagobert D., ed. 2007. *The Selected Writings of Benjamin Rush*. New York: Philosophical Library.

Rush, Benjamin. 1790. *Enquiry into the Effects of Spirituous Liquors on the Human Body*. Boston: Thomas and Andrews.

———. 1798. *Essays: Literary, Moral and Philosophical*. Philadelphia: University of Pennsylvania.

Sassatelli, Roberta, and Alan Scott. 2001. "Novel Food, New Markets and Trust Regimes: Responses to the Erosion of Consumers' Confidence in Austria, Italy and the UK." *European Societies* 3, no. 2: 213–44.

Saxton, Rufus, quoted in Edwin D. Hoffman. 1956. "From Slavery to Self-Reliance: The Record of Achievement of the Freedmen of the Sea Island Region." *Journal of Negro History* 41: 8–42.

Schlesinger, Arthur. 1947. "A Dietary Interpretation of American History." *Proceedings of the Massachusetts Historical Society* 3, no. 68: 199–227.

Schlosser, Eric. 2011. *Fast Food Nation: The Dark Side of the All-American Meal*. New York: Houghton-Mifflin.

Schulten, Susan. 2013. "A Capitalist Case for Emancipation." *Opinionator, New York Times,* February 6. http://opinionator.blogs.nytimes.com/2013/02/06/a-capitalist-case-for-emancipation.

Sears, Clara Endicott, ed. 1915. *Bronson Alcott's Fruitlands with Transcendental Wild Oats, by Louisa M. Alcott*. Boston: Houghton Mifflin.

Seldes, Gilbert. 2012. *The Stammering Century*. New York: NYRB Classics.

Severson, Kim. 2007. "For U.S. Food Elite, an Unlikely (Crowned) Hero." *New York Times,* April 25.

———. 2007. "Lunch with a Food Revolutionary: Don't Worry, She'll Bring the Capers." *New York Times,* September 19, F1.

————. 2008. "Slow Food Savors Big Moment." *New York Times,* July 23, F1.

Shanahan, Fergus. 2002. "Probiotics and Inflammatory Bowel Disease: From Fads and Fantasy to Facts and Future." *British Journal of Nutrition* 88, no. 1: s5–s9.

Shapiro, Laura. 2001. *Perfection Salad.* New York: Random House.

Shprintzen, Adam D. 2013. *Vegetarian Crusade: The Rise of an American Reform Movement, 1817–1921.* Chapel Hill: University of North Carolina Press.

Shulman, Martha Rose. 2009. "Collard Greens: Rethinking a Southern Classic." *New York Times,* October 26. www.nytimes.com/2009/10/26/health/26recipehealth.html.

Sinha, Mrinalini. 1995. *Colonial Masculinity: The "Manly Englishman" and the "Effeminate Bengali" in the Late Nineteenth Century.* New York: Manchester University Press.

Smith, Andrew, and Bruce Kraig. 2012. *The Oxford Encyclopedia of Food and Drink in America,* vol. 1. New York: Oxford University Press.

Spencer, Charles. 2008. *Edisto Island, 1861 to 2006: Ruin, Recovery and Rebirth.* Charleston, SC: History Press.

Spencer, Herbert. 1860. "The Social Organism." *Westminster Review* 73, no. 143: 90–121.

————. 1981 [1884.] *The Man versus the State, with Six Essays on Government, Society and Freedom.* Edited by Eric Mack, with an introduction by Albert Jay Nock. Indianapolis: LibertyClassics. Accessed May 3, 2015, http://oll.libertyfund.org/titles/330.

Stahr, Walter. 2012. *Seward: Lincoln's Indispensable Man.* New York: Simon & Schuster.

Sullivan-Fowler, Michaela. 1995. "Doubtful Theories, Drastic Therapies: Autointoxication and Faddism in the Late Nineteenth and Early Twentieth Centuries." *Journal of the History of Medicine and Allied Sciences* 50: 364–90.

Swyngedouw, Erik. 2010. "Apocalypse Forever? Post-political Populism and the Spectre of Climate Change." *Theory, Culture and Society* 27, nos. 2–3: 213–32.

Tarr, Joel. 1996. *The Search for the Ultimate Sink: Urban Pollution in Historical Perspective* Akron, OH: University of Akron.

Tauber, Alfred I. 1994. *The Immune Self: Theory or Metaphor?* New York: Cambridge University Press.

Taylor, Charles. 1994. "The Politics of Recognition." In *Multiculturalism: Examining the Politics of Recognition,* 25–71. Princeton, NJ: Princeton University Press.

Taylor, Joe Gray. 1982. *Eating, Drinking and Visiting in the South: An Informal History.* Baton Rouge: Louisiana State University Press.

Taylor, William R. 1963. *Cavalier and Yankee: The Old South and American National Character.* New York: Doubleday.

Thomas, John L. 1965. "Romantic Reform in America, 1815–1865." *American Quarterly* 17, no. 4 (Winter): 656–81.

Titus, Mary. 1997. "The Dining Room Door Swings Both Ways: Food, Race and Domestic Space in the Nineteenth Century South." In *Haunted Bodies: Gender and Southern Texts,* edited by Anne Goodwin Jones and Susan V. Donaldson. Charlottesville: University Press of Virginia.

Tocqueville, Alexis de. 2002 [1835]. *Democracy in America*. Penn State Electronic Classics Series. University Park: Penn State University Press.

Tomes, Nancy. 1997. *The Gospel of Germs: Men, Women, and the Microbe in American Life*. Cambridge, MA: Harvard University Press.

Tompkins, Kyla Wazana. 2012. *Racial Indigestion: Eating Bodies in the 19th Century*. New York: New York University Press.

Trees, Andrew S. 2003. *The Founding Fathers and the Politics of Character*. Princeton, NJ: Princeton University Press.

Tucker, Todd. 2006. *The Great Starvation Experiment: Ancel Keys and the Men Who Starved for Science*. Minneapolis: University of Minnesota Press.

Vandergeest, Peter. 1996. "Real Villages: National Narratives of Rural Development." In *Creating the Countryside: The Politics of Rural and Environmental Discourse,* edited by E. Melanie DuPuis and Peter Vandergeest. Philadelphia: Temple University Press.

Vanloqueren, Gaetan, and Phillipe Baret. 2009. "How Agricultural Research Systems Shape a Technological Regime that Develops Genetic Engineering But Locks Out Agroecological Innovations." *Research Policy* 38, no. 6: 971–83.

Verbrugge, Martha H. 1988. *Able-Bodied Womanhood: Personal Health and Social Change in Nineteenth-Century Boston*. New York: Oxford University Press.

Viet, Helen Zoe. 2013. *Modern Food, Moral Food: Self-Control, Science and the Rise of Modern American Eating in the Early Twentieth Century*. Chapel Hill: University of North Carolina Press.

Vos, Timothy. 2000. "Visions of the Middle Landscape: Organic Farming and the Politics of Nature." *Agriculture and Human Values* 17, no. 3: 245–56.

Wald, Priscilla, Nancy Tomes, and Lisa Lynch. 2002. "Introduction: Contagion and Culture." Special Issue. *American Literary History* 14, no. 4 (Winter).

Wallace, William, and Christopher Phillips. 2009. "Reassessing the Special Relationship." *International Affairs* 85, no. 2: 263–84.

Watson, Duika Burgess, Tiago Moreira, and Madeleine Murtagh. 2009. "Little Bottles and the Promise of Probiotics." *Health* (London) 13, no. 2: 219–34.

Whatmore, Sarah, and Lorraine Thorne. 1997. "Nourishing Networks: Alternative Geographies of Food." In *Globalising Food: Agrarian Questions and Global Restructuring,* edited by David Goodman and Michael Watts, 287–304. London: Routledge.

White, Philip. 2012. *Our Supreme Task: How Winston Churchill's Iron Curtain Speech Defined the Cold War Alliance*. New York: Public Affairs.

Whorton, James C. 2000. *Inner Hygiene: Constipation and the Pursuit of Health in Modern Society*. New York: Oxford University Press.

Wiebe, Robert H. 1966. *The Search for Order, 1877–1920*. New York: Hill and Wang.

Williams-Forson, Psyche A. 2006. *Building Houses Out of Chicken Legs: Black Women, Food, and Power*. Chapel Hill: University of North Carolina Press.

Wood, Gordon S. 2009. *Empire of Liberty: A History of the Early Republic, 1789–1815*. New York: Oxford University Press.

Young, Iris Marion. 2000. *Inclusion and Democracy.* New York: Oxford University Press.

Young, James Harvey. 1989. *Pure Food: Securing the Federal Food and Drugs Act of 1906.* Princeton, NJ: Princeton University Press.

Zahari, Lofty. 2008. "Dannon Activia Yogurt and Bifidus Regularis." *M. D. O. D.,* April 14. http://docsontheweb.blogspot.com/2008/04/dannon-activia-yogurt-and-bifidus.html.

INDEX

American Founders. *See* Founding-Era America; *specific individuals*

American Physiological Society, 44

The American Woman's Home (Beecher and Stowe), 55, 63, 65

Animal, Vegetable, Miracle (Kingsolver, Kingsolver, and Hopp), 101, 102

antebellum reform movements, 21, 29–53; embrace of vegetarianism, 36–37, 40–42, 43–44, 53; and European culture, 44–45; and the industrializing economy, 33–34, 35; influence on later social movements, 52–53; as moral endeavors, 30–32, 33, 42, 49; overviews, 10, 29–30, 52–53; rejections of mainstream values, 10, 29–30, 31–32, 35; romanticism and, 10, 29–30, 32, 33, 38, 43, 51; self-improvement focus, 31–33, 52–53; Southern rejection of, 45–50; use of the press, 33; utopian experiments, 40, 50–53; views of Southern culture and politics, 30, 35. *See also* abolitionism; civic romanticism

Anthony, Susan B., 43

Anti-Slavery Society, 29

Appadurai, Arjun, 147

aristocracy and aristocratic ideals, 9, 18, 22, 30, 45, 109

The Art of Right Living (Richards), 81

Asian diets and foodways, 69–71, 88–90, 91, 105, 108

Atkinson, Edward, 35, 61, 62, 64, 68, 70

Atwater, W. O., 67–69, 70, 170n47

Aurora Dairy, 132–33, 135

autointoxication, 84–85

autonomy, 9, 17, 18, 19, 20, 73

bacteria: soil microbes, 145. *See also* fermentation; germs; metabiome; probiotics

Baden-Meyer, Alexis, 124

Battle Creek sanatorium, 83

Baudrillard, Jean, 98

Beecher, Catharine, 48, 65; *The American Woman's Home* (Beecher and Stowe), 55, 63, 65

Beecher, Harriet. *See* Stowe, Harriet Beecher

Beecher, Henry Ward, 65

beneficial bacteria. *See* metabiome; probiotics

beri-beri, 88

Berlin Wall, 1, 4

Berry, Wendell, 102

Bifidobacterium, 142

"Bifidus Regularis," 142

bifurcations, 1–4, 6–7, 111–12, 148, 161n3; as the enemy of progress and reform, 7–8, 10–11; the nature/culture bifurcation, 111, 113, 145–46; the purity/danger bifurcation, 2, 5, 32, 112, 118. *See also* boundaries; purity

Billings, C. K. G., 72

Bittman, Mark, 98

Black Hunger (Witt), 161n3

the body: medical views of, 21; Progressive-Era notions of the ideal body, 79, 87, 91; reimagining embodiment, 12; the skin as boundary, 139; as social/political metaphor, 6, 7, 75–77, 78, 83. *See also* fermentive ecologies and politics; metabiome

Bosch, Laurentine ten, 115, 117

Boston Cooking School, 66, 81

boundaries and boundedness, 12, 13, 137, 161n3; boundary-work, 112, 113–15, 149; and the national organic standards process, 124, 125–26, 128, 130; and Progressive hygiene ideology, 78, 83–84, 87, 113; and romanticism in the modern alternative food movement, 110

Bourdieu, Pierre, 113

Bove, Jose, 106

Breakthrough project, 111–12

Brisbane, William Henry, 62

Brook Farm, 50

Brown, John: the Harpers Ferry raid, 35, 41

Brown, Valerie, 153

Bruni, Frank, 105

Buck, J. L., 89–90

Buck-Morss, Susan, 7

Burned-Over District, 39; Rochester as a locus of reform, 41–43

Cullen, William, 21
Current Literature, 70
Curtis, Jamie Lee, 140–41
Cyborg Manifesto (Haraway), 161n3

dairying and dairy foods: in an agroecological system, 158–59; dairy-centered diets seen as superior, 88, 89, 90–91, 93; as key to Northern agriculture and diets, 66, 72, 88, 93; McCollum's work promoting milk drinking, 90–93; milk drinking, 40, 88, 89, 90–91, 93; the NOSB's Organic Pasture Rule, 131–33; yogurt, 85, 140–42, 143
DanActive, 141
danger, 145; the purity/danger bifurcation, 2, 5, 32, 112, 118. *See also* purity and purification
Danone/Dannon, 85; probiotic yogurts, 140–42, 143
Davis, David Brion, 18
Deans Foods, 135
Debs, Eugene, 69, 70
decision-making processes, for wicked problems, 153–54, 157–60. *See also* fermentive ecologies and politics
degeneracy: diet and, 93; eugenics and, 86; Southern culture and values stigmatized as, 30, 35, 58, 65–66. *See also* self-indulgence; temperance
Democracy in America. See Tocqueville, Alexis de
Democratic Party, 30, 34, 49
detoxification, 112, 114, 115–19; enemas, 73, 85
dichotomies. *See* bifurcations
didacticism: civic republican, 20–21, 33; in modern alternative food movements, 100–101, 102, 103, 117, 147, 151; in nineteenth-century reform movements, 33, 35–36, 40–41, 42, 51, 55; in the Progressive Era, 81
"diet," etymology of, 5–6
dietary advice and reform, 5–6, 7–8, 11; antebellum reformers, 31–32, 36, 39–44, 50–52; antebellum Southern rejection of, 45–49; in Founding-Era America, 17,

23; in post–Civil War America, 55–57, 66–69, 73, 74; in Progressive-Era America, 78, 80–85, 87–94. *See also* modern alternative food movements; nutrition science; temperance; vegetarianism; *specific periods of American history*
"A Dietary Interpretation of American History" (Schlesinger), 71–72
digestion: the human microbiome, 138–39, 142–43, 145–46; immunity and, 139, 142; as metaphor, 12, 145, 157; Metchnikoff's work, 84–85; probiotics, 85, 139–43
digestive subjectivity, 12, 145–51. *See also* fermentive ecologies and politics
DiMatteo, Katherine, 127
The Discovery of France (Robb), 107
disease: dietary deficiency diseases, 63, 88, 130; foodborne illness and its prevention, 119–24, 122*fig.,* 177n21; germs and contagion, 10, 77–78, 113; Graham on Cholera, 44; immunity, 83–84, 139, 142; martial narratives of, 143; the Mediterranean Diet and, 104; studies on heart disease and diet, 105. *See also* health; hygiene and sanitation ideologies
Dixon, Bernard, 118
Douglas, Mary, 2
Douglass, Frederick, 43
Dr. Strangelove, 159–60
dualisms. *See* bifurcations
Durkheim, Emile, 75, 76
dyspepsia products, 73

E. coli outbreaks, 119–20, 122*fig.*
Eat Right and Stay Well the Mediterranean Way (Keys and Keys), 105
Eat Well and Stay Well (Keys and Keys), 105
ecology: the human metabiome as an ecosystem, 138–39, 142–43, 145–46; Leopold on predator management, 144–45. *See also* agroecology; fermentive ecologies and politics
economic inequality, 91, 99; poverty viewed as sin, 43. *See also* inequalities

economics: industrialists and
nineteenth-century Northern
reformers, 33–34, 35, 54; modern diets
and, 99–100, 101; Progressive-Era
anxieties about, 78–79; traditional
European rural cultures and, 107; wages
and wage struggles, 53, 67–71, 86, 89,
100. *See also* efficiency; elite; home
economics; industrialization; middle
class; working class
Edisto Island, 59, 60*fig.*
efficiency, economic and nutritional, 55–56,
67–70, 76, 82
elimination. *See* exclusion/elimination
elite consumption practices, 10, 66, 72
elitism: abolitionism and vegetarianism
seen as elitist, 37; the modern
alternative food movement seen as
elitist, 108
Ely, Richard, 86
Emerson, Ralph Waldo, 29, 32–33, 36, 42,
50, 51
enemas, 73, 85
"Enquiry into the Effects of Spirituous
Liquors" (Rush), 23, 24*fig.*
EPIC (European Prospective Investigation
into Cancer and Nutrition), 104
equality, 25, 27
Erie Canal, 39, 41, 43
Ernst, Edzard, 118
ethnic foods and diets, 104–5; as
model healthy diets, 108; seen as
inferior/unhealthy, 69–71, 88–90,
91, 100
eugenics, 83, 85–87; "euthenics" as an
alternative to, 81, 83, 86–87
European culture: the American Founders'
views of, 22; and the antebellum middle
class, 44–45; European Romanticism,
10, 29–30, 38, 43, 45, 51. *See also*
aristocracy
European foodways, 66, 104, 105; the
Mediterranean Diet, 104–6, 107–8;
modern food movements' sacralization
of, 103–10, 147; S.A.D. in Europe, 106;
Slow Food and, 103–4
European immigrants. *See* immigrants and
immigration

European Prospective Investigation into
Cancer and Nutrition (EPIC) study,
104
euthenics, 81, 83, 86–87
evangelism: civic-romantic embrace of,
38–39
exclusion/elimination, 7–8, 145, 149, 160;
racial exclusion policies, 69–70, 93. *See
also* boundaries

fair trade, 159
fast food, 72, 98, 101, 106
FDA (Food and Drug Administration),
FSMA implementation by, 114, 119, 120,
123–24
Federalist Papers, 19
feminist scholarship, 6
fermentation: digestive, 143; as metaphor,
12, 13, 14, 146–51, 157
fermentive ecologies and politics, 138–60;
characteristics of, 145–46, 147–48,
149–50; the human metabiome, 138–39,
142–43, 145–46; and the potential for
social change, 146–47, 148, 149–51,
157–60; probiotics, 85, 139–43;
tolerating danger and wildness, 144–45;
wicked problems and new solution
processes, 152–57
fiber, 98, 118
Finney, Charles Grandison, 38–39, 40,
41–42, 43–44
Fisher, Irving, 80, 82, 83
Fitzpatrick, Frank, 108–9
Fletcher, Horace, 80, 82–83
Florida, Harriet Beecher Stowe's work in,
62–63, 65
Food, Inc., 102
Food, Morals and Meaning (Coveney), 17
Food and Drug Administration. *See* FDA
food choices: bifurcated narratives of, 2–3,
4; moral views of, 9. *See also specific
geographic, ethnic, and social groups*
Food Matters (film), 115
Food Revolution, 97
food revolution. *See* modern alternative
food movement
food safety: Hartley's campaign against
unsanitary dairies, 40

food safety/purity, 12, 13, 114, 137;
foodborne illness outbreaks, 119–23,
122*fig.*, 177n21; the Food Safety
Modernization Act, 114, 119,
120, 123–24; Progressive-Era activism
and reforms, 78, 79–80, 82,
87, 93
A Fool's Errand (Tourgée), 65
FOS (fructooligosaccharides), 130, 131
Foucault, Michel, 6
Founding-Era America, 9, 17–28; civic
republicanism and freedom as self-
control, 5, 9, 18, 19, 20–21, 27, 33;
freedom as property ownership,
19–20, 25, 26–27, 30, 34; the
freedom/order tension, 18, 19; free
labor and small producer narratives,
34–35, 37, 49, 61, 63; the Hamiltonian
view of freedom, 19, 20; overviews, 9,
17–18, 25–28; Rush's writings, 21–25,
24*fig.*; slavery in, 9, 19–20
Francis, Coni, 130
Franklin, Benjamin, 19, 20
Freakonomics, 120
Freedmen's Bureau, 61, 62, 63
freedom ideologies and narratives, 1–5;
freedom as individual autonomy, 19;
freedom as property ownership,
19–20, 25, 26–27, 30, 34, 42; freedom
as self-control, 9, 18, 19, 20–25, 27, 33.
See also autonomy
free labor narratives, 34–35, 37, 49, 61, 63
free will. *See* autonomy
French diets and foodways, 104, 106
French Revolution, 22, 29
French Women Don't Get Fat, 104
fructooligosaccharides (FOS), 130, 131
Fruitlands, 50–51, 115
FSMA (Food Safety Modernization Act),
114, 119, 120, 123–24
Fugitive Slave Law, 49
functional foods, 130–31
Funtowicz, Silvio, 153–54
Furstenberg, François, 27

Galton, Francis, 86
GAP (good agricultural practice)
programs, 120

Garrison, William Lloyd, 32, 34, 35, 38, 41,
42. *See also* Anti-Slavery Society
Garvey, T. Gregory, 52
gastro-tourism, 108–9
Gaytan, Sarita, 103
Genovese, Evelyn Fox, 48
George IV of England, 26*fig.*
germs and contagion, 10, 77–78; foodborne
illness and its prevention, 119–24,
122*fig.*, 177n21. *See also* disease; hygiene
and sanitation ideologies
Gerstle, Gary, 149
"Gideon's Band," 59–60
Gieryn, Thomas, 112
Gilded-Age America. *See* post-Civil War
America
Gillray, James, 26*fig.*
Gilroy, Paul, 161n3
Gliesmann, Steve, 133
gluttony, 23. *See also* overeating;
self-indulgence
Godey's Lady's Book, 37
the golden mean, 79
Gompers, Samuel, 69–70, 70–71
good agricultural practice (GAP)
programs, 120
Good Health (magazine), 83
Good Housekeeping, 82
Good Morning America, 104
Graham, Sylvester, 36, 40–41, 42, 43–44,
102, 165n47
Grahamite boardinghouses, 44, 45
Graham Journal of Health, 44
Graubard, Barry, 101
Greeley, Horace, 35, 36–37, 41
greens, 91–93, 106, 147
Grimke, Angelina, 41
Grimke, Sarah, 41
The Guardian, 118
Gudstadt, Herman, 69–70
Gullah culture and communities, 63

HACCP (Hazard Analysis and Critical
Control Points) programs, 120
Hagan, Key, 120
Hale, Sarah Josepha, 37, 47
Hall, Stuart, 8
Hamilton, Alexander, 19

Haraway, Donna, 161n3
Harding, T. Swann, 89
Hardman, W. B., 87
Harpers Ferry raid, 35, 41
Hartley, Robert, 40
Harvey, Arthur, 124, 126, 131
Haskins, Sarah, 142
Havel, Vaclav, 4
Hazard Analysis and Critical Control
   Points (HACCP) programs, 120
health: ethnic diets seen as
   unhealthy/inferior, 69–71, 88–90,
   91, 100; Graham's ideas about, 36;
   health impacts of the S.A.D., 3, 118; and
   the Mediterranean Diet, 104–5;
   Metchnikoff's work on immunity and
   digestion, 83–85; Progressive-Era
   notions of, 79, 83–84; Progressive-Era
   public health initiatives, 78, 79, 83,
   84fig.; Rush's views on temperance,
   21–25, 24fig.; self-indulgence viewed as
   unhealthy, 22–23, 25, 36. See also
   disease; hygiene and sanitation
   ideologies; nutrition science
health claims: health criteria in the NOSB
   process, 130–31; for probiotics, 140–41,
   142
heart disease, diet and, 105
Heasman, Michael, 98, 99
Hecker, Isaac, 51
hedonism. See pleasure; self-indulgence
History of Nutrition (McCollum),
   91–92
HIV, 143
Hoard's Dairymen, 91
Hobbes, Thomas, 19
Hofstadter, Richard, 19
Holmes, Oliver Wendell, 86
home cooking, 101. See also cooking
home economics, 55, 68, 78, 80–82
Hopkinson, James, 59, 60fig.
Horizon Dairy, 135
hospitality, 47–48
housekeeping: household hygiene and
   sanitation, 77–78. See also cooking;
   home economics
How to Live (Fisher), 82
Human Gut Microbiome Initiative, 138

human metabiome, 138–39, 142–43,
   145–46. See also digestion; fermentive
   ecologies and politics
Human Metagenome Project, 138
Hunt, Lynn, 17
Hurston, Zora Neale, 64
hybrid collectivity, 146
hybridity: vs. bifurcations, 2, 161n3. See also
   fermentive ecologies and politics
hygiene and sanitation ideologies, 113, 151;
   anti-immigrant policies and, 71; clean
   eating narratives, 117; cleanliness as
   health, 80; disease and, 10, 77–78, 113;
   eugenics and, 86–87; foodborne illness
   and, 119, 123; and the human
   microbiome, 139, 145–46; Leopold on
   the sanitizing of wilderness, 144–45;
   overviews, 10, 77, 113; personal
   detoxification, 112, 114, 115–19; in the
   Progressive Era, 10, 77–78, 80–85, 86,
   87, 113. See also food safety

ideals and idealism, 7–8, 10, 11. See also
   perfectionism/Perfectionism;
   romanticism/Romanticism
immigrants and immigration, 10, 12, 42–43,
   49, 86; Chinese diet seen as a threat to
   American workers, 69–71; immigrant
   dietary attitudes and aspirations, 66–69,
   71–72, 73; the industrial food system's
   reliance on immigrants, 99; racial
   exclusion policies, 69–70, 93. See also
   ethnic foods; working class; working-
   class diets; specific immigrant groups
immunity: digestion and, 139, 142;
   Metchnikoff's work, 83–84
Imperial Leather (McClintock), 161n3
inclusiveness: inclusive problem-solving
   processes, 156–58. See also exclusion
Indian diets, 88, 91
individualism, 18. See also autonomy
industrialization and industrial interests:
   and post–Civil War cotton agriculture
   in the South, 60–61; post–Civil War
   wage and diet tensions, 53, 67–71;
   worker efficiency and nutritional
   efficiency, 55, 67–70, 76, 82. See also
   organized labor; working class

Martin, Emily, 143
Massachusetts Reconstruction Association, 62
mastication, 82–83
masturbation, 23, 44
materialism: among the emergent working class of the mid–nineteenth century, 34–35, 49; rejections of, 36, 46–47. *See also* pleasure; self-indulgence
McClintock, Anne, 161n3
McCollum, E. V., 90–93
McDonald's, 106
meat eating, 10, 66; in anti-abolitionist newspaper rhetoric, 37; as key to Northern diets, 72, 88; Rush's views on, 22, 23, 25; by the working class, 56, 66–71. *See also* Northern diet(s); plant-based diets; vegetarianism
meat production, 3, 99, 100
media: abolitionism in the antebellum press, 36–37, 41, 165n30; Chinese lifestyles in the nineteenth-century press, 70; civic republicanism and the press, 20–21; detoxification practices in, 117–18; foodborne illness coverage, 120; modern food reformers in, 101–2, 104, 105–6, 109; Northern antebellum reformers' use of, 33; in the Progressive Era, 78, 79–80, 81, 82, 88–89. *See also* advertising; literature; *specific publications*
"A Medical Essay on Drinking" (O'Flaherty), 24*fig.*
medicine. *See* disease; health; Rush, Benjamin
Mediterranean Diet, 104–6, 107–8
Mediterranean Harvest: Vegetarian Recipes for the World's Healthiest Cuisine (Shulman), 106
Mélard, François, 157
Mellosi, Martin, 113
metabiome, human, 138–39, 142–43, 145–46. *See also* digestion; fermentive ecologies and politics; probiotics
Metchnikoff, Elie, 80, 83–85
Mexican foodways, 100, 105, 108
miasmas, 77

microbiome, human. *See* digestion; fermentive ecologies and politics; metabiome, human
middle class emergence and values, 42–43, 44–45, 54, 100. *See also* antebellum reform movements
milk drinking, 40, 88, 89, 90–91, 93. *See also* dairying and dairy foods; Northern diet(s)
milk production, 131–33, 158–59. *See also* dairying
Miller, William, 39
minimum-wage policy, 89
Minnesota Semi-Starvation experiments, 105
moderation. *See* temperance
modern alternative food movements, 11, 97–110; didacticism in, 100–101, 102, 103, 117, 147, 151; embrace of the Mediterranean Diet, 104–6, 107–8; Eurocentrism in, 103–10; hypocrisy and elitism charges, 108; moral and romantic dimensions of, 100–103, 106–7, 109–10, 150; overviews, 11, 97–100, 109–10; the S.A.D. and its critics, 3, 97–100, 108, 110; Slow Food, 99, 103–4, 106, 107, 108–9. *See also* organic food
Molnar, Virag, 113
moralism and moral values, 4, 10, 17; in antebellum reform movements, 10, 30–32, 33, 35–36, 42, 49; in the modern alternative food movement, 100–102, 150. *See also* self-control; virtue; Yankee virtue
Morgan, Edmund, 19, 20
Mormon Word of Wisdom, 39
Morton, Timothy, 43
muckraking journalism, 78, 79–80, 82

national character, diet equated with, 69–71, 88–89
National Health Interview Survey, 101
National List of Allowed and Prohibited Substances, 124, 126, 128–31. *See also* National Organic Standards Board
National Organic Program (NOP), 125

National Organic Standards Board (NOSB) process, 124–36; background, 124–26; and consumer expectations, 125; as a discursive process, 112, 114–15, 128–30; diversity of actors and interests, 126–28, 134; functional foods and the use of health criteria, 130–31; ingredients emphasis, 131; large-scale/corporate actors and, 127, 129, 130, 132–33, 135, 136; the Organic Pasture Rule, 131–33; public input and debate, 127, 128–29, 130, 131–32, 133–36; small-scale/noncorporate actors and, 125, 126–27, 132

nature: the modern alternative food movement's embrace of, 103, 104, 106–7; the nature/culture bifurcation, 111, 113, 145–46; Romantic and civic-romantic embrace of, 10, 30, 33, 43–44. *See also* Romanticism

New Deal, 149

New England Kitchen, 68, 73, 81

New England reformers. *See* abolitionism; antebellum reform movements

"New England Reformers" (Emerson), 32–33

The Newer Nutrition (McCollum), 90–91

New York Cooking School, 66, 81

New York Herald, 36–37, 165n30

New York Times, 105, 108–9

New York Tribune, 36–37, 165n30

NOP (National Organic Program), 125. *See also* National Organic Standards Board (NOSB)

Northern culture and values: Southern foodways as resistance to, 56. *See also* antebellum reform movements; civic republicanism; Yankee virtue

Northern diet(s): as the American Ideal, 72, 118; equated with social and physical superiority, 88–92, 93; immigrant rejection of, 73. *See also* American diet(s); Standard American Diet

Northern reformers: and agriculture restructuring in the post–Civil War South, 59–63, 64; missionary efforts in the post–Civil War South, 62–63, 65; the Port Royal Experiment, 59–62, 64–65; post–Civil War missionary endeavors among African American

freedmen, 59–60, 62–63. *See also* abolitionism; antebellum reform movements; *specific individuals*

NOSB. *See* National Organic Standards Board

nutraceuticals, 130–31

nutrition science: Keys's work, 105; modern nutrition advice, 97–98; nineteenth-century applications of, 67–69, 73; nutritionists' current embrace of the Mediterranean Diet, 104–5; in the Progressive era, 76, 79, 82–85, 87–93

nutrition transition, 98. *See also* Standard American Diet

Obama, Barack, 119

Oberlin College, 40

obesity and overweight, 97, 98, 106. *See also* overeating

O'Flaherty, Thomas, 24*fig.*

Oliver, Jamie, 97

The Omnivore's Dilemma (Pollan), 103, 109–10

Oneida community, 40

order, 9, 12, 17, 18, 22

organic foods and agriculture, 99, 100–101, 159; label requirements, 125; strawberry production manual development process, 154–56. *See also* National Organic Standards Board

Organic Foods Production Act, 124–25

Organic Trade Association (OTA), 127

organized labor, 69–71, 76, 89

Orientalism (Said), 161n3

OTA (Organic Trade Association), 127

overeating, 23, 56, 57*fig.,* 73–74, 115

Oz, Mehmet, 117

Paltrow, Gwyneth, 117

Parsonnet, Julie, 139

pasta, 107–8

Pasteur Institute, 85

patent medicines, 56, 57*fig.*

Paulist Fathers, 51

pellagra, 63

perfectionism/Perfectionism, 7–8, 10, 31–32, 38–39, 52–53. *See also* ideals and idealism

Perishable Pundit, 123
personal transformation. *See* self-improvement; self-purification
Petrini, Carlo, 106, 108, 109
Philbrick, Edward, 61, 62
Pickering, Andrew, 5
plant-based diets, 108; ethnic diets as, 100, 104–5, 108; the Mediterranean Diet, 104–6; stigmatization of, 88, 91–93, 100, 104–5. *See also* vegetarianism
pleasure: the pleasure/self-control tension, 27, 56; as unhealthy, 22, 23, 25. *See also* materialism; self-indulgence
Poe, Edgar Allen, 46
Poison Squad, 82
politics: antebellum reformers and, 29, 31, 32, 35, 36–37, 49–50, 53; party politics of the 1840s, 49–50; the Progressive outlook on, 79–80. *See also* civic republicanism; fermentive ecologies and politics
Pollan, Michael, 98, 99, 103, 108, 109–10, 126
pollution, 115, 117. *See also* detoxification; purity
Popkin, Barry, 98
pork, 58, 105, 106
Port Royal Experiment, 59–62, 64–65
Post, C. W., 73–74
post–Civil War America, 54–74; class and diet-related struggles, 66–69, 72–73; high-consumption habits and the emergence of commercial antidotes, 56, 57*fig.*, 73; overviews, 10, 54–58; race and diet-related struggles, 58–65, 69–72; Southern agricultural restructuring and land redistribution, 58–65; the stigmatization of Southern foodways, 65–66
post-normal science, 153–54, 159
poverty: viewed as sin, 43. *See also* inequalities
"The Powers of Horror" (Kristeva), 161n3
press. *See* media; *specific publications*
Prevor, Jim, 123
print culture. *See* literature; media; *specific authors and publications*
probiotics, 85, 139–43

processed foods, 97, 98–99. *See also* industrialized food; Standard American Diet
Progressive-Era America, 80–94, 112; anthropometrics and the ideal body, 79, 87; eugenics, 83, 85–87; Fisher's work on calories, 82; Fletcher and mastication, 82–83; hygiene ideologies and narratives, 10, 77–78, 80–85, 86, 87, 113; Kellogg and the Battle Creek sanatorium, 83, 87; Metchnikoff's work on immunity and digestion, 83–84; overviews, 10, 76–80, 93–94; race and ethnicity and nutrition reform, 87–94; Richards and home economics as a profession, 55, 78, 80–82; Wiley and the Poison Squad, 78, 80, 82, 83, 86, 87
The Prolongation of Life (Metchnikoff), 84–85
property ownership: and the emergence of the middle class, 42; as an ideology of freedom, 19–20, 25, 26–27, 30, 34, 42; land redistribution in the post–Civil War South, 61–62, 63–64; rejections of, 51
protective foods, 85, 90, 92
public health initiatives, Progressive-Era, 78, 79, 84*fig.*, 87; "euthenics," 81, 83, 86–87
Pure Food and Drug Act of 1906, 78, 82, 87
purification treadmills, 11, 94, 111–12, 136, 157; the Food Safety Modernization Act as, 114; organic standard setting as, 114–15, 125; personal detoxification, 115–19; utopian endeavors as, 50. *See also* confoundings/conundrums; food safety; National Organic Standards Board (NOSB) process
Purity and Danger (Douglas), 2
purity and purification: eugenics as social purification, 86; problems with purity politics, 6–8, 10–11, 13–14, 115, 136, 157; as Progressive ideal, 77, 78, 80, 83, 87, 93–94; the purity/danger bifurcation, 2, 5, 32, 112, 118. *See also* food safety; hygiene and sanitation ideologies; purification treadmills; self-purification

race and race relations: diets equated with racial inferiority, 69–71, 88–90, 92–93; racial exclusion policies, 69–70, 93; racial nationalism, 149. *See also* African Americans; immigrants and immigration; slavery

race betterment, 86. *See also* eugenics

Race Betterment Foundation, 83, 87

race suicide, 86

Racial Indigestion (Tompkins), 6, 7, 161n3

Ravetz, Jerome, 153–54

The Raw and the Cooked (Levi-Strauss), 2

Reagan, Ronald, 4

Reconstruction, 55, 61, 63, 65; land redistribution and agriculture restructuring in the occupied South, 59–65. *See also* post–Civil War America

reflexivity, 135–36, 149, 150, 156, 158

religion. *See* spirituality

Republican Party, 34

resistance, 10, 13–14, 27; African American freedmen and the restructuring of Southern cotton agriculture, 58–65; class and race-related dietary struggles in post–Civil War America, 54–56, 66–73; to Northern antebellum reform efforts, 34, 36–37, 47–49

restaurant meals, 101

revelation and revelation narratives, 39–40, 103, 117, 140

Revolutionary America. *See* Founding-Era America

Reynolds, David, 30–31

rice-centered diets, 69–71, 88–90, 91, 93, 108

Richards, Ellen Swallow, 68, 70, 73, 78, 80–82, 86

Riddle, Jim, 128–29, 130

Robb, Graham, 107

Roberts, Robin, 104

Rochester, New York, 41–43

romanticism/Romanticism, 7–8; antebellum reform movements and, 10, 29–30, 32, 33, 38, 43, 51; in modern food reform movements, 101, 102–3, 106–7, 109–10; and the NOSB Organic Pasture Rule, 131–32, 134–35; in probiotics

advertising, 140–41. *See also* civic romanticism

Roosevelt, Theodore, 79–80

Ross, Edward, 86

Rousseau, Jean-Jacques, 29

Rush, Benjamin, 19, 20, 27, 32, 36; writings of, 21–25, 24*fig.*

Rush, John, 25

Said, Edward, 161n3

salads, 92

Salmonella outbreaks, 122*fig.*

A Sand County Almanac (Leopold), 144–45, 180n17

Sanger, Margaret, 87

sanitation. *See* hygiene and sanitation ideologies

Sargent, Dudley, 79

Saturday Evening Post, 88

Savard, Marie, 104

Saxton, Rufus, 59, 61, 62, 168n17

Schlesinger, Arthur, 71–72

Schlosser, Eric, 98

Schneider, Keith, 120

science and scientific analysis: centrality for the Progressives, 76–77; efficiency analysis, 55–56, 69; nineteenth-century reform movements and, 10, 40, 43–44, 54, 55; post-normal science for wicked problems, 153–54; rise of the professional expert, 77, 80; scientific boundary-work, 112; tacit knowledge and, 155–56. *See also* nutrition science

Scott, Walter, 30, 46

Sea Islands communities and agriculture, 59–62, 63, 168–69n21

self-control/self-denial/self-discipline, 3, 5, 6; of Chinese immigrants, 69–71; commercial products as alternatives to, 56, 57*fig.*, 73–74; freedom as, 9, 18, 19, 20–25, 27, 33; the pleasure/self-control tension, 27; in the rhetoric of modern food reform, 100–101; utopianism and, 40, 50–51. *See also* self-indulgence; temperance; Yankee virtue

self-improvement: Perfectionism, 38–39; reformers' faith in, 31–33, 52–53

CALIFORNIA STUDIES IN FOOD AND CULTURE

Darra Goldstein, Editor